Public Health Advocacy
Creating community change to improve health

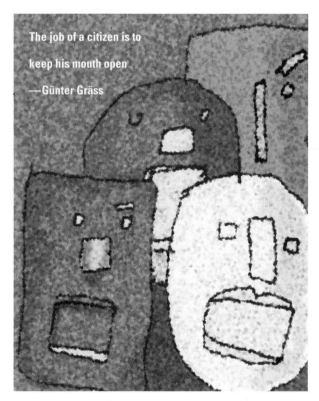

The job of a citizen is to keep his mouth open
—Günter Grass

David G. Altman
Stanford University

Fabricio E. Balcazar
University of Illinois

Stephen B. Fawcett
University of Kansas

Thomas Seekins
University of Montana

John Q. Young
Stanford University

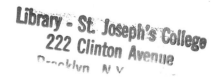
STANFORD CENTER FOR RESEARCH IN DISEASE PREVENTION
IN COOPERATION WITH THE KAISER FAMILY FOUNDATION

Stanford Center for Research in Disease Prevention
1000 Welch Road, Palo Alto, CA 94304-1885

Public Health Advocacy was developed under a grant from
the Henry J. Kaiser Family Foundation, Menlo Park, CA

The mention of trade names, commercial products or organizations does not imply endorsement by
Stanford University, nor by the funder of this project.

ISBN 1-879552-12-4

Book design: Eunice Ockerman

Contents

Acknowledgements

The authors would like to acknowledge the generous support of the Henry J. Kaiser Family Foundation, without which this project would not have been completed.

We would also like to thank the staff at the Stanford Health Promotion Resource Center for their constant support and encouragement while this handbook was being written. We are especially grateful to Ellen Feighery and Juliette Linzer for their contributions, and to Marcia Jarmel for her editorial assistance.

Richard Olive, Karen Peterson, Vince Francisco and Adrienne Page provided editorial assistance on various chapters. Richard, in particular, helped to translate our original ideas into a more readable form.

Finally, Prudence Breitrose, editor extraordinaire, played a key role in making the manual organized, cohesive and accessible.

Note: At intervals throughout the handbook, quotations are included from anonymous advocates with the following organizations: The Department of Health and Hospitals, Boston, Mass.; The Partnership for Democracy, Portland, Ore.; Families, USA, Washington, D.C.; The Sierra Club (Bay Area Chapter), Oakland, Calif.; Health Care for All, Boston, Mass.; The Harvard School of Public Health, Cambridge, Mass.; and The American Association of Retired Persons, Washington, D.C. Our thanks to the advocates and their organizations.

Introduction

Youth violence. Homelessness. Teenage pregnancy. Drug use. Drinking and driving. Nicotine addiction. AIDS. Air and water pollution. Mushrooming health care costs, and uneven access to medical care. Increasingly, problems like these have spurred individuals to become advocates—to speak out and get involved in community health issues through active citizen participation.

The goal of this handbook is to foster the growth of public health advocacy. To this end, we will take you through the entire process, from the first vision to the final evaluation, with plenty of examples showing how advocacy strategies and tactics are actually being applied by community health professionals and citizen activists.

One of the challenges in writing a handbook on public health advocacy is to make it usable, so it doesn't end up gathering dust on the bookshelf. By combining a general overview with practical "how-to" material, we hope to motivate health workers and grassroots organizers to put the ideas and techniques we have presented into practice. It is said that people remember 20 percent of what they hear, 40 percent of what they hear and see, and 80 percent of what they discover for themselves. We hope that most readers will end up in the 80 percent group—discovering how to apply the material in their communities, and adapt it to their needs.

The audience

Both seasoned advocates and newcomers to advocacy should find useful material. Readers might include health educators working for local or state government, health professionals and paraprofessionals working with community-based organizations, grassroots community organizers and volunteers, professionals working in community-based health promotion organizations, and members of community-health coalitions. For lack of a better term, we call the individuals participating in the advocacy process *community health activists*.

Overview of Handbook Contents

This handbook is dedicated to the "how," and will focus on tools and solutions. Its objective is to give confidence to newer advocates and restore excitement, joy and vigor to some war-weary veterans. Specifically, we begin with preparatory steps, including the development of a vision for change, then progress through questions of leadership, organization of your own group, and outreach into the community. Next follows practical advice on researching an issue, and analyzing it in order to select the most effective points for intervention.

Once you know what you want to do, the question is, "how"? The center of the book provides hints on the "etiquette" of advocacy tactics, and worksheets that you can use to clarify your own ideas on specific objectives and ways to reach them. After a chapter on strategic planning, tactical advice follows, with specific tactics to suit your own needs, and suggestions for turning the opposition's counter-tactics to your advantage. Following this, you will find a chapter that helps you use the media effectively and constructively, and another with hints on evaluating your efforts. Finally, we include case-histories that illustrate how the advice in this handbook can be applied in practice.

We don't intend to dwell too much on the definition of issues, but will concentrate on finding solutions. As you work through the material presented, keep in mind the following perspective:

- You are not alone in your desire and efforts to right wrong;
- The bad news of hopelessness looms *much* larger than its actual size;
- If your aim is to challenge those people, places or things that are damaging to community health, you can make a difference.

Those new to public health advocacy may have the advantage of an open mind as they approach the content of this handbook. You will be free to pick your way through the various approaches and tactics, choosing what's best suited to the issue, the community, and your style.

More experienced advocates may be tempted to skim over the ideas presented here, since they are familiar to you. However, we urge you to take another look. You may find that the handbook enables you to try a fresh approach, taking you out of the cycle of "doing the same things over and over while expecting different results!"

1

First Steps in Advocacy: The Vision

Public health advocacy involves efforts to change community conditions related to health. It's David against Goliath, consumers against commercial giants, families against polluters, citizens fighting city hall, parents protecting their children from harm, and public-spirited groups seeking access to health services for those who cannot fend for themselves.

Some people believe that community health advocacy is synonymous with confrontation and conflict. Although conflict is sometimes unavoidable, effective activists know when and how to cooperate just as well as when and how to confront—they use the democratic process. Indeed, community activism is rooted in the democratic principles and practices that have characterized this nation since its inception—the democratic spirit that De Tocqueville (1840) remarked upon in his observations of American customs in the nineteenth century.

Community health advocacy involves the *active* espousal of a cause or principle, and *actions* that lead to a goal considered worthwhile by the people involved. Here are some examples:

- The coalition in that steered an ordinance through the local political machinery to get cigarette machines banned in San Jose, California;
- The group of parents who advocated successfully for the removal of asbestos from public schools in their community;
- The saga of Love Canal in New York, beginning when one homemaker, Lois Gibbs, focused attention on the relationship between a toxic waste site and the high incidence of miscarriages and low-birthweight infants in the area.

The growing need

There has always been room for advocacy, but in recent years the need has become greater as the emphasis in health promotion and disease prevention has shifted. We no longer think solely in terms of encouraging individual behavior change—exhorting the smoker to quit, the drinker to stay off the road, or the parent to provide nutritious food. We realize that all of these goals can be achieved faster and better if changes are also made in the environment, through adjustments to policies, laws, or the expected social norm.

In some cases, these environmental changes will provide back-up for individual behavior change—for instance, when improved labels enable people to make more healthful food choices. In other cases, advocacy for environmental change becomes the prime weapon—for example, when it provides protection against second-hand smoke, or ensures that laws against drunk drivers are enforced.

Who are the advocates?

There are many reasons why people join advocacy organizations or become involved in advocacy activities. In some cases, they are drawn into action by some personal experience, especially one that is negative or traumatic. For example, having a child with a disability, or a family member who gets lung cancer from smoking, can be the salient event that propels people into action. Indeed, many health advocacy organizations were developed because an individual or a small group of people decided to take action—such as Mothers Against Drunk Driving, founded by Candy Lightner after her own daughter was killed.

Health advocacy organizations exist at the professional level, where advocates such as lobbyists, workers in voluntary health agencies, and union officials earn their living advocating for others. This handbook, however, is geared to grassroots efforts for health advocacy—efforts that are organized and conducted largely by volunteers, perhaps under the direction of a small (under)paid staff.

"What keeps an advocate going? In my case, a lot of it is what I see in individuals I work with—watching them get empowered. It gives me a bedrock faith in people."
AN ADVOCATE

The vision

Health advocacy groups that can articulate a shared vision are more likely to be successful than groups that wander from issue to issue without a clear focus or mission. A vision articulates the types of changes you would like to bring about. It is your view of how the community would look and function if all was well. Ultimately, a vision is the creative force that drives a health advocacy effort, and attracts the support of the critical mass of people whose backing may be essential to your success.

Developing the vision

In essence, the vision is a broad statement of the reason your group exists. It provides an important tool for the organization and leadership of your group, in the following ways:

- A vision helps recruit and organize a group. It can be used to show the commonalties of individual experiences. ("I see that you are shocked by youth violence—you are not the only one who wants a safe and healthy neighborhood!")
- A vision can be used to justify a group to others, by explaining in broad and general terms the need for change and the changes needed. ("I'll tell you why we're here! We stand for peace in the neighborhood"). It is both an important public education tool and a device to protect you from attack, enabling you to justify your positions and actions.
- A vision can help guide important decisions by your group, bringing you back to the basic purposes the group shares. ("Let's remember why we started this. We may disagree about tactics, but we all want to create a community that is good for our children.")

Within the context of community health advocacy, a vision transforms isolated personal experiences into a shared focus for change. For example, the parents of a young child who is injured by schoolyard violence may feel their family is the victim of an unfortunate but isolated event. With this perspective, they may become confused and depressed, because the school administration seems indifferent to growing violence, and the parents feel they have nowhere to turn. They may withdraw their children from public school, and, at enormous cost, put them in a private school, which they feel will be safer.

Alternatively, if the parents know of other such incidents, or talk with other parents whose children have been injured, their experience may be transformed from the isolated personal event to one that provides a shared focus on change. The group that forms around this common sense of outrage may develop the strength to challenge the school administration, and encourage it to take measures to protect the children.

The ideal vision has five important features:

1. A vision statement captures an ideal state.
"Health for all." "Healthy adolescents." "Peace in the neighborhood."
These vision statements capture a broadly held ideal.

> "Get a very clear vision and stick with it, but reassess your vision at every step—take in new information and use it to make your vision more attainable."
> AN ADVOCATE

2. **A vision promises to address a shared problem.**

   The problem may be one that people have experienced directly, such as the loss of a loved one in an automobile collision caused by a drunk driver. It may also be one that affects the advocates less directly, such as teen pregnancy.

3. **The vision defines the conditions that can and should be changed.**

   For advocacy to be effective, the main cause of the problem must lie *outside* the individuals affected, residing instead in some element of their circumstances. For example, the advocate is unlikely to have an effect on the behavior of a drunk driver, who may or may not choose to stop drinking after a fatal crash. However, advocates can approach the problem by way of the circumstances outside the drinker, which may include:
   - Lack of enforcement of alcohol sales and driving laws;
   - Insufficient education about drunk driving in the public school system;
   - The portrayal of alcohol consumption as glamorous in the media.

   Thus, in this case, the vision might suggest the need to improve and enforce alcohol consumption laws, to provide better alcohol education in the public schools, and to change the media portrayal of alcohol use. In essence, those who begin an advocacy group—whether it is started by one person or a group of like-minded activists—will need to describe the broad agenda for changes that they envision in a way that others can relate to.

4. **A vision helps convey the notion of both personal responsibility and personal capacity.**

   For example, in recruiting parents to join an anti-drunk driving campaign, you might say, "We have the energy for this. The lives of our sons and daughters are at stake. Who will take responsibility to act, if we don't?"

5. **Finally, a vision conveys hope, and suggests the possibility of success.**

   This involves showing a personal commitment to action (e.g., "I'm in it for the long haul.") It also involves explaining the reasons you believe things can be improved.

As your group grows and starts the long process of planning a campaign, you may find yourselves enmeshed in debate about specific decisions. In such instances, it is vital to have a clear view of the visionary roots that underlie the purpose of your group. We've all been in meetings where two or more factions of the same group were in a heated and seemingly unresolvable debate, when someone said something like, "Wait a minute. Can we go back to why we're doing this in the first place?" Recalling the original vision can keep the discussion on target, and foster cooperation and team unity. When the group feels frustrated or down because of an apparent failure, returning to the vision is like going back to the well for a drink of cool water on a hot day. It refreshes and rejuvenates. Talking about it can re-build a sense of hopefulness, optimism, and the possibility of change for the better, through your efforts.

Creating the vision

Suggestions for creating the vision are in Chapter 5, where you will find worksheets to help you consolidate your strategic plans for the campaign, including the vision, the mission and the objectives.

A personal statement: our own vision

It would be unfair to expect you to develop a clear statement of your personal vision without expecting the same of the authors. Our own vision is one of safe and healthy communities for all. We believe that individual citizens, working together, can be effective in changing community conditions. We have all been a part of such efforts, and have been witness to dozens of others.

What we saw, individually at first and then collectively later, was that many people who wanted to take charge of events in their communities lacked ideas about how to begin. Once they got started, the situation provided its own guidance; it was getting off on the right foot that was difficult.

We believe we can make a difference by joining with others in our communities to attack common health concerns such as drug abuse, violence, inaccessible health care, diseases caused by pollution and poverty, or social problems brought on by ignorance and unhealthy lifestyle choices. Other communities have succeeded in improving their health by taking the kind of action described here. We believe you can make that difference, too.

2

Building Your Group

In this chapter, we will discuss some of the factors involved in starting a grassroots advocacy group, including its membership, its leadership, and its contacts with other agencies, institutions or organizations in the community.

Starting an advocacy group

A group may be started when one or two people realize the need to initiate advocacy, and get others who share their vision to join in the effort at hand. You may identify people who share your concerns simply by listening to what they say about their experiences. For example, you may hear people complaining of their difficulty in gaining access to local social services, or expressing their concern about their children's exposure to drugs. If these concerns are similar to those you feel yourself, or are shared by others whom you know, you can initiate a connection, and suggest that something be done about the problem.

For many people, making contact can be embarrassing, especially if the need to start an advocacy group springs from something that has personal implications—for example, if it involves a health problem that affects someone in your family. However, you will often find that others are grateful that you have made contact.

The time to make this contact is when your desire for action is fresh, and you encounter someone else who is also currently concerned about the issue. Here are some suggestions for that first approach:

- Tell people how you are affected by the issue.
  For example: "My daughter was hit by a drunk driver, too."
- Tell them what you see as the problem.
  For example: "Drug pushers shouldn't get away with selling to our kids."
- Describe the important values you feel are being threatened by the status quo.

For example: "None of us feel secure when violence is outside one person's door."

- Explain how you think that, together, you can make a difference. For example: "If we stick together, we can make this a safe neighborhood."

If there seems to be interest, organize a meeting of like-minded people, or invite them to a regular meeting if your group is already formed.

Making your approach

The first impression that you make on people you approach can have a significant effect on their attitudes, and their willingness to join in your project. Here is a checklist you can use as you embark on your recruitment (adapted from Speeter: *Power: A Repossession Manual*):

- Do I seem open to people about why I am organizing?
- Am I clear about my purposes?
- Am I clear about my methods? Do I propose solutions as well as problems and questions?
- Are the issues I am raising too threatening? If so, how can I make them less threatening?
- Is my appearance threatening? Does it undermine my credibility?
- Is my manner threatening? Do I talk more than I listen?
- Do I convey feelings in a way beneficial to the project?

Involving others

One of the most important principles of community health advocacy is that you should include many representatives of the community in your efforts—not just members of a small clique. By training others, you will not only aid the growth of individuals, but build the human resources of the community itself. People who experience success and satisfaction by working with your program are more likely to tackle other community issues and concerns later on. In a word, you are helping to build leaders.

If advocacy is to be *with* people and not *for* them, the people who are personally affected by the health concern must be involved. An environmental toxic waste campaign would involve neighbors of the toxic dump. A teen pregnancy prevention effort would involve adolescents. A youth violence initiative would involve youth at risk to gangs, and their parents.

There are many other individuals and groups you may want to include as allies in your advocacy efforts, such as health care providers, teachers, school principals, religious leaders, and business people. In considering those who might be drawn to your effort, you need not be overly concerned with conflicts between people. (Working on the same side of an issue may even bring them together!)

Leadership

Leadership comes about in many different ways. A leader might be the person who first articulates the vision and forms an action group to try and bring it to fruition. Or the leader might emerge after the group has come together. In some cases, the leader will play a dominant role, coordinating the efforts of group members, directing operations, taking charge of planning, or supervising the execution of a plan of operations. In other cases, a leader may be expected to delegate much of the planning and operation of an organization's activities to others, and be involved only in setting broad goals and resolving disputes through his or her decision-making authority.

In some groups, leadership may be shared. Or indeed, leadership may be seen as the efforts of *any* member of a group to take the initiative. It is this leadership role that every member can play, but that only a few take on at any one time. Broad-based, diverse leadership can be an important resource, providing the type of group dynamic that imparts a purpose, goal, dream or vision to others, and conveys a sense of hope and optimism for the future.

The hallmark of effective leadership is often not so much skill in management as the ability to provide a vision that others can carry out. Leaders should also be able to adapt a leadership style to the variety of contexts in which action is required. This flexibility is often an overlooked skill.

The leaders' roles

Leaders need to maintain the energy of the group, and motivate members by conveying a sense of hopefulness, optimism, and possibility for success. Here are some tips to help keep members' activities focused on important efforts, and their interest and energy high (more can be found in the publications listed in "Additional Resources" on page 161):

- Plan activities that do not exceed the capacity of members to achieve them;
- Plan for enough time, support and resources to accomplish tasks;
- Plan for many successes, rather than aiming for one goal that may prove impossible to attain;

"A leader should be someone who understands that the process of getting people's input is as important as the outcome...
It doesn't take a lot of time to be a dictator. It takes a lot of time to be process oriented."
AN ADVOCATE

- Acknowledge group accomplishments and individual achievements;
- Acknowledge personal achievements (although this may best be done privately).

Maintaining group unity

The best reward for members of a group is often purposeful work, followed by a sense of accomplishment: work itself may provide the glue you need to turn your group into a cohesive force. The middle chapters in this handbook will help you to achieve a sense of satisfaction through a systematic process of research and planning. The later sections of the book provide the tactics and actions that can lead to actual progress in your advocacy campaign, and the satisfaction that comes from achievement. Meanwhile, your shared vision will give you strength and cohesion that can carry you over the times when things do not seem to be progressing well.

Involvement in a community of interest—people who share the same concerns—is empowering. Members committed to a cause are strengthened by knowing they are not alone—that they share a mission. It is also a relief to know that, in the final analysis, the campaign does not rise or fall on individual strength and weakness. However, advocacy can bring its own brand of stress to groups engaged in it. As you will see in later chapters, the group may be faced with choices with the potential to be divisive—decisions about strategy and tactics, decisions that may involve antagonizing people of influence in the community, or even decisions about civil disobedience.

A strong, democratically run group united in its cause is best suited to survive the ups and downs of wins, losses and crises. The keys to a group's unity may lie in the strength of the organizational structure, the availability of channels for active participation, and a clear focus on goals. The organization's strength will be shored up significantly if there is individual accountability among the members, with a common awareness that they are responsible to each other and the group, and must be ready to account for their actions. It is particularly important that group members learn they can rely on the leadership. A leader accustomed to shooting from the hip or flying solo is likely to be viewed as a "troublemaker" or as damaging to the group in some other way.

Self-discipline by each member strengthens the group's ability to persist in the face of repression. It cannot be imposed. Gene Sharp, in *The Politics of Nonviolent Action*, says self-discipline provides not only for growth on the part of the activist, but for internal strength that can earn the respect and recognition of others, both within and outside of the group.

Collaboration with other groups

As we proceed through the sections of this handbook that deal with planning and implementing your advocacy actions, we will remind you as appropriate to consider the need for community involvement in your campaign. It is important for the long-term health of the community that you use existing resources, or build new ones with community help, rather than simply importing ideas, programs or materials from the outside.

You may find that other groups or agencies are already trying to reach the same people in the community. Whether you are currently in agreement with these groups on all aspects of the issue or not, collaboration can prove fruitful. Cooperative arrangements offer an excellent way to expand limited resources, and present a powerful image to the community. Working together can bring the maximum available force to bear on the opposition.

Suppose, for example, that you want to persuade the city council to pass an ordinance protecting non-smokers from passive smoke. You are more likely to be effective if spokespeople from several groups are included among those making presentations. There is a down side, however. Once other groups step in, complete with their own agendas, compromise is sometimes necessary. (Also, practical matters such as scheduling meetings for all interested parties may become much more difficult.) On the plus side, by working together you will have greater resources for accomplishing difficult tasks. Your group's reputation for cooperation on important community issues will be enhanced, and the potential visibility of the issue, and perhaps of your group, will be increased. If leaders of other groups endorse your program, it may also increase the chances of grassroots community support.

In the next chapter, you will find hints for identifying potential allies, as your advocacy group conducts research into your chosen issue.

"When spider webs unite,

they can tie up a lion."

ETHIOPIAN PROVERB

Lessons from Geese

Taken from a talk by anthropologist Angeles Arrien
(as printed in the newsletter of the Maryland Association
of Extension Home Economists).

Fact 1

As each bird flaps its wings, it creates an uplift for the bird following. By flying in a **V** formation, the whole flock adds 70 percent greater flying range than if one bird flew alone.

Lesson 1

People who share a common direction and sense of community can get where they're going quicker and easier because they're traveling on the strength of one another.

Fact 2

Whenever a goose falls out of formation, it suddenly feels the drag and resistance of trying to fly alone, and quickly gets back into formation to take advantage of the lifting power of the bird immediately in front.

Lesson 2

If we have as much sense as geese, we will stay in formation with those who are ahead of where we want to go, and be willing to accept their help as well as give ours to others.

Fact 3

When the lead goose gets tired, it rotates back into formation and another goose flies the point position.

Lesson 3

It pays to take turns doing the hard tasks and sharing leadership.

Fact 4

The geese in formation honk from behind to encourage those up front to keep up their speed.

Lesson 4

We need to make sure our honking from behind is encouraging, and not something else.

Fact 5

When a goose gets sick or wounded or shot down, two geese drop out of formation and follow it down to help and protect it. They stay with it until it is able to fly again or dies. Then they launch out on their own, or join another formation.

Lesson 5

If we have as much sense as geese, we, too, will stand by each other in difficult times as well as when we are strong.

3

Understanding the Issue

In this chapter, we will introduce you to some of the tools that can help you prepare a solid factual base for advocacy.

We will start by encouraging research into the broader context for your advocacy actions. Next, we will give suggestions for ways to document your issue. Finally, the chapter provides techniques to help you find the basic causes of the problem you are addressing, and hence the best point for intervention.

Understanding broader trends

Conducting research into broader trends can be helpful in ensuring that you are not missing anything important that may affect your issue, now or in the future. If you can anticipate change, you are less likely to be disoriented by it, and more likely to understand where you can most efficiently direct your energies.

Three broad trends are particularly important to consider, because change is occurring in these fields so rapidly. These are the information age; globalism; and cultural diversity.

1. The information age

Members of your group should keep abreast of changes in communications technology because these changes may affect the way we conduct our advocacy campaigns. For example, if interactive cable television allows two-way communications on public issues, knowledge of its potential could affect your choice of tactics.

2. Globalism

As with the information age, keeping abreast of trends in the global village can help you find appropriate targets for your actions, and guide you in your choice of strategy and tactics.

Many problems that were once local are in fact now also global. The proliferation of pesticides is an example. Banning local application of a dangerous chemical won't do your community much good if local markets are selling imported produce sprayed with the same substance. Conversely, you might achieve a local victory at the expense of a distant disaster. For example, if you succeed in banning toxic dumping in your region, you may be sentencing the population of a part of Africa to the same danger, since multinational corporations sell "dump markets" in areas that don't have restrictive policies.

3. Cultural diversity

Awareness of other cultures is increasingly important. Our society is no longer a "melting pot" where ethnic minorities are assimilated into the dominant white culture. We are a "salad bowl" of many ethnic communities that are holding onto their identities and cultural values. As we embrace this diversity, our health promotion focus will be increasingly multi-cultural, making our advocacy efforts more relevant to the growing variety of our communities. Specifically, two types of questions should be addressed:

Questions of sensitivity:
How representative of the community is your group? Is it culturally sensitive? How culturally specific will your advocacy efforts be? Will you use language, metaphors, and expressions which the community of interest understands and feels comfortable with?

Questions of responsiveness:
Do your group's issues address needs of minority communities, or only needs perceived by the majority society? Are your advocacy efforts responsive to the interests of diverse communities?

How to track broad trends

There are several resources helpful for identifying and following those three important trends. The United Way of America regularly publishes a book, *What Lies Ahead*. Two magazines also feature articles on megatrends: *Future Survey* and *The Futurist*.

To an extent, of course, this background research will be informal—a matter of keeping up with the newspapers, monitoring talk shows, and listening to what people are saying. To make sure that no major developments are missed, we suggest that you designate members of your group to make this type of research a formal part of their regular routine.

Getting down to specifics

In order to plan and carry out effective advocacy action, you will need to be thoroughly familiar with your chosen issue and its effect on your community—understanding its history, its economic effect, the people involved, the extent to which they are affected, the political background, and so on. Nothing can sink an advocacy group faster than being caught with its facts wrong, or incomplete. Conversely, if you are knowledgeable about all aspects of the issue, you will not only be in an excellent position to choose appropriate strategies and tactics, but your mastery of facts will earn the respect of the community, the media and even the opposition.

Some members of your group might be impatient at the prospect of delay while you conduct research. They may even quote Martin Luther King, Jr.'s caution about the "paralysis of analysis." It is important, however, to make it clear to the group that this next stage in the planning process is essential if you are to base your program on a solid foundation.

The questions

Here is a list of questions in different categories that may serve as a starting point for your research:

Who is affected by the issue?
- Who is affected most?
- Who loses? How so?
- Who gains? How so?

What are the consequences of the issue?
- What are the consequences for the individuals most affected?
- For their families?
- For society?

What is the economic impact of the issue?
- What are the economic *costs* of this issue? Who bears these costs?
- What are the economic *benefits* of this issue? Who benefits?

What are the barriers?
- What are the barriers for addressing this issue?
- How can they be overcome?

What are the resources?
- What are the resources for addressing this issue?
- Where can they be tapped?

"There are no quick solutions. What is needed is a lifetime commitment, acknowledging that we are in a continuing revolution and revelation, and that the means cannot be separated from the ends any more than an individual may be separated from the community."
LILLIAN AND GEORGE WILLOUGHBY, *PEACE CALENDAR*

What is the history of this issue?
- What is the history of the issue in the community?
- What past efforts were made to address it?
- What was the result?

Documenting the issue

The word "documenting" should not be interpreted too narrowly. Your aim is not simply to amass facts and data, but to find out how people in your community feel about the issue; where the important community leaders or other players stand on it; and what are the potential ramifications for the business community, the legal system, the health care system, the school system, or local government.

Research will continue throughout the life of your advocacy project, but it is especially important in the beginning. If your background knowledge is incomplete, or you make factual mistakes, this will give a huge advantage to any opponent—as you will see when you reach Chapter 4, "Advocacy 'Etiquette'," Chapter 7, "Advocacy Tactics," and Chapter 8, "Dealing with the Opposition."

Throughout the project, imagine yourselves in debate with your opponents. Imagine the hardest questions that might be thrown at you. Make sure that you have the answers right at your fingertips.

Here are some sources that members of your group might use to find specific information:

The local media

The local newspaper can be an excellent source of information. While news stories can keep you abreast of developments in relation to your issue, letters to the editor may offer insight into the way people feel about it. Local radio talk shows may also serve as a barometer of feeling or resentment about local problems. One advantage of these shows is that you can sometimes call in yourselves, and guide the debate. (See Chapter 9 for ideas on using the media.)

Organizational newsletters; minutes from board meetings

Depending on the nature of your issue, newsletters or minutes of meetings may provide valuable information. (See Chapter 7 for tactics that involve using these means to gain an edge in your dealings with specific opponents.)

Issue papers, study reports, annual reports

Many organizations issue reports that are publicly available, even though they may be filed away, never to be used. You may have to dig around to get these reports, but they are often worth the effort, revealing positive or negative changes in policy, unmet needs, or hostile actions which might relate to your group's mission.

Existing surveys

Check to see if any other group in your community has completed a recent survey that you can use. Your United Way, health department or city government might know which groups have similar interests to yours, and which might have conducted research.

Archival records

A look at formal records may give you the information you need. For example, factual information from law enforcement records, court records, school records, and records from health and human service agencies is all available. Your local reference librarian may be of help in this phase of the search.

This is the way one advocate used existing records to build his case:

Michael Bennet, a Michigan pipefitter, became aware of an apparently high incidence of cancer deaths among fellow workers. Bennet spent two years reviewing death certificates of local workers to compare cancer frequency with the national rate. He found twice as many cases of lung cancer as would have been predicted from the national experience. While Bennet's study did not determine the cause of this higher local incidence, it left no doubt that a problem existed. (See Legator, Harper, & Scott: *The Health Detective's Handbook.*)

Doing your own research

In cases where the information you need has not been collected by anyone else, you could initiate your own data collection. This may require professional help, but that need not be expensive. Often advocates within health departments and other local agencies may be able to help you, contributing skills and experience. You may be able to carry out simple data collection without outside help; the materials listed in "Additional Resources" on page 161 can give you guidance. We will briefly describe four types of data collection: the community resource inventory, the community leader survey, the community opinion survey, and the focus group. Using more than one method will increase your understanding of the issue, and your confidence in knowing that you have identified a need that deserves your energy, and are laying a firm foundation for your campaign.

The community resource inventory

A resource inventory can tell you what community groups are currently working on your issue, or are potentially interested in your issue—and what capacity exists for additional facilities and services. Sometimes a resource inventory will be done to help you find whether resources are available to meet specific needs. Sometimes it can go beyond that, and lead you to potential allies, collaborators, coalition partners, or sources of help. For example, if you are interested in curbing youth violence, you might find a parent group that is also engaged in an advocacy program. By collaborating with the other group, rather than competing, you can maximize the resources of both. The United Way and other local agencies may be aware of inventories that list resources within federal, state, city or private organizations. Even if they don't provide the specific information you want, these inventories can provide a good starting point.

Community leader survey

This type of survey involves seeking out key leaders, exploring their attitudes to your issue, learning from their specialized knowledge, and listening to their suggestions for solutions. Leaders may include people in a position to control resources or make decisions, or they may simply be respected members of the community, with no official position. Often, one can suggest others who will be helpful. Be cautious in approaching any leaders who might be opponents of your advocacy actions, because you may not want to alert the opposition at this early stage to the fact that you are organizing. When you approach leaders who are sympathetic to your cause, on the other hand, interviews may open the way to collaboration.

Community opinion survey

This type of survey allows you to collect information directly from members of the community, documenting specific health needs, health-related behaviors, knowledge and beliefs. Similar surveys conducted before and after a campaign can be used to evaluate that campaign, and provide evidence of change. Such surveys should not be undertaken lightly, however; they require expertise in identifying a representative sample of the population; phrasing questions; and analyzing responses. (See "Additional Resources" on page 161 for more information.)

Focus groups

Groups of eight to twelve members of the community—meeting for one to two hours under the guidance of a skilled moderator—can help you probe attitudes and beliefs, and test out ideas for actions or programs. You may need to conduct multiple groups to make sure you are hearing from all relevant sections of the community.

What next?

When you have completed your basic research into the issue, you may be drowning in facts, opinions and data. Your next task is to continue the research process by identifying the basic cause of the problem, which will help you find the most fruitful point of intervention.

Analyzing possible causes

Analyzing causes will help you to do the following:
- Select that part of an issue that is most amenable to change;
- Find where change will have the best effect;
- Identify the "stakeholders"—those who benefit from the way things are, and those who will benefit from change;
- Identify "targets of change" (those who contribute to the problem);
- Identify "agents of change" (those who can contribute to a solution).

Here is an example: in addressing the issue of teen pregnancy, a group's first instinct is to suggest education of the girls themselves. Digging deep to find the cause, however, they find that education isn't what is needed. Rather, the increase in births can be traced to the closure of the school clinic that dispensed contraceptives, and to the lack of prospects for good jobs. As a "target of change," the group then identifies the school principal, who has led the opposition to a school clinic. An "agent of change" might be the local Chamber of Commerce, which could be persuaded to provide more job opportunities for youth.

In other words, careful causal analysis can save you from the mistake of oversimplifying an issue, and help you apply your efforts in a way that will have the most effect. As another example, consider two different ways of approaching a problem in a school where a handful of children with severe behavior problems are disrupting classroom routine:

Solution 1
You lobby the school district to hire extra "special education" teachers.

Solution 2
Analyzing the causes of the disruptions, you find that a high proportion of these youngsters are suffering from Fetal Alcohol Syndrome (FAS). You may choose to

continue with your plans for the hiring of special teachers, but you may also decide to put much of your energy into stopping the flow of FAS children into the school system in the first place. You find out what makes the mothers drink; you arrange for them to have education or treatment; you lobby for better display of warning notices in liquor store.

The river analogy

Causal analysis is a way to "look upstream" at societal problems, as illustrated in this story:

One day, as a man was fishing from a river bank, he saw a youth being swept downstream, struggling to keep his head above water. The man dived in, grabbed the youth, and struggled with him to shore. The youth thanked the man and went on his way, and our hero dried himself off and returned to his fishing. But shortly he heard another cry, and saw a woman being swept downstream. He jumped into the river again, and saved her. And that went on all afternoon. As soon as our hero got back to his fishing again after saving someone, he would hear another cry, and haul out another wet and drowning person. Finally he said to himself: "Before I kill myself trying to save drowning people I'd better go upstream and find out who's pushing them in."

Catching the problems upstream

It may be helpful (staying with the river analogy) to consider each issue in terms of midstream, downstream and upstream questions. With each potential issue that you face, we suggest that you ask yourself these questions, and do the research necessary to find the answers.

Downstream questions:
What is the effect of this issue on the community?
What is the effect on related health issues?

Midstream questions:
What is the health issue or concern?
Who has a need for change or help?

Upstream questions:
What causes the health concern?
What needs to be done upstream to prevent the problem,
or at least make it less serious?

"There are a thousand hacking at the branches of evil to one who is striking at the root ..."
HENRY DAVID THOREAU,
WALDEN

How to conduct an analysis of root causes

There are numerous techniques for analyzing root causes. We will describe one.

The "But why?" method

David Werner, a community health organizer in Latin America, developed the "But why?" method of identifying and understanding root causes. In his case, this method was useful for coming to grips with the causes of wide-spread ill health among villagers in western Mexico:

[At first] I did not look far beyond the immediate causes of ill health. As I saw it, worms and diarrhea were caused by poor hygiene and contaminated water. Malnutrition was mainly caused by scarcity of food in a remote, mountainous area where drought, floods, and violent winds made farming difficult and harvest uncertain. Little by little, I became aware that many of their losses—of children, of land or of hope—not only have immediate physical causes, but also underlying social causes ....There is a photograph of a very thin little boy in the arms of his malnourished mother. The boy eventually died—of hunger. The family was—and still is—very poor. Each year the father had to borrow maize from one of the big landholders in the area. For every liter of maize borrowed at planting time, he had to pay back three liters at harvest time. With these high interest rates, the family went further into debt. No matter how hard the father worked, each year more of his harvest went to pay what he owed to the landholder.
   —Werner: *Helping Health Workers Learn*

The "But why?" method used by Werner can help advocates avoid incorrect or inadequate analysis of issues, and thus prevent the wasteful misapplication of strategies and tactics.

Here's how it works. A group examines a health problem by asking what caused it. Each time someone gives an answer, the group asks, *"But why?"* Here is one simple example offered by Werner:

Downstream issue
The child has a septic foot.
But why?

Midstream issues
Because she stepped on a thorn.
But why did she step on a thorn?
Because she has no shoes.

But why doesn't she have shoes?
Because her father can't afford shoes for her.
But why?

Upstream issues
Because he is a poor farm laborer.
But why?

And so forth. Here's another example of the "But why?" process and the issues it can yield, this time addressing the problem of access to tobacco products by minors:

Downstream issue
Children get cigarettes easily from stores and vending machines.
But why?
Because merchants don't know about laws governing illegal tobacco sales.
But why don't they know about these laws?

Midstream issues
Because police have not enforced existing laws.
But why?
Because there is a perception that other drug use and crime are more important community issues.
But why aren't tobacco problems considered important?

Upstream issues
Because the tobacco industry has succeeded in framing tobacco issues to their advantage.
But why hasn't the issue been framed differently?

And so forth.

After you have exhausted all "But whys?" you can decide which answers and issues represent the best possible points of intervention. If you find points of intervention on many different levels, so much the better. If resources allow, intervention on multiple levels will be more effective than simply on one.

The "But why?" technique can be applied to the exploration of either individual or societal root causes:

1. It can be used to find which *individual* factors could provide targets of change for the advocate, such as levels of knowledge, awareness, attitudes, and behavior:
   - Do people need more knowledge about nutrition?
   - Do children need to learn refusal skills, to avoid smoking?
   - Do teenagers need to learn how to use contraceptives?

2. It can explore *social* causes, in three main sub-groups:
- Cultural factors such as customs, beliefs, and values;
- Economic factors such as those related to money, land, and resources;
- Political factors such as decision-making power.

Refining the choice of targets

In the process of documenting your issue, and asking "But why?" you have probably found targets for change—perhaps too many! Some targets may simply turn out to be impractical, or aiming for them may not be cost-effective. In addition, the list of potential targets will probably be narrowed down and refined through the processes that follow in this book, especially the sections on selection of objectives and strategy. However, there are two additional methods of identifying targets for change that you might want to apply at this stage to make sure you are exploring all possibilities: *Conversations with key decision-makers*, and *Power structure research*. Both of these methods involve going to the top. As you will see, the difference between them is largely one of degree—the first is relatively informal, while the second can be quite demanding, time-consuming and potentially hazardous to the health of your project.

In both cases, these words of warning apply: Approaching people who might prove to be targets of your advocacy action at an early stage brings obvious hazards. If done clumsily, these approaches could alert those in power of your impending action. They could in turn take measures that would discredit you early; deflate your potential tactics; close doors that you would prefer remain open. What follows here should be applied with extreme care—and not before you have read through later chapters in this book, especially "Advocacy 'Etiquette'" (Chapter 4) "Advocacy Tactics" (Chapter 7) and "Dealing with the Opposition" (Chapter 8).

In both of these approaches, you will be seeking answers to these two questions:

1. **Who are the potential targets of change?**
   Who is responsible for the problem? Whose behavior contributes to the problem?

2. **Who are the potential agents of change?**
   Who has the power to solve the problem? Or whose behavior could contribute to a solution?

Conversations with key decision-makers

This method of isolating targets for change simply involves interviewing decision-makers, and attempting to find out from them who has the power. This can be very informative—but it is not an action to be undertaken lightly, especially in the early stages, before you are ready for confrontation with those who might oppose you. It bears repeating that if you need to interview someone who may turn out to be a target of your advocacy, you should use great care.

- Suppress the urge to reveal all that you know about the issue and your informant's role in it.
- At this stage, your goal is to listen and learn—not to confront, nor to commit yourself to any action.
- Once you have interviewed an individual, use him or her to gain access to the next person. Then, as you move along the chain of influence you can say, "So-and-so suggested you'd be an important person to talk to."

Power structure analysis

Power structure analysis is a more formal process, helping you search for points of intervention all the way up to the top of an organization, agency or governmental body. Here are two sample situations in which these techniques can be helpful:

1. You have identified a factory's waste disposal methods as a health hazard in your community, and you have expressed concern to the company several times. Time and again you are passed from one person to another. How do you find the source of power in the company, and apply appropriate pressure?
2. A program of the local health department geared toward controlling tobacco use seems to ignore high-risk segments of the community. You have not had any success talking to program implementers in the local agency offices. How do you identify and reach the decision-makers?

Those with the power to make change are not always easy to identify. Information is the key to identifying the doors they can be found behind, and to unlocking these doors.

You can start in a very positive manner, with the attitude that, "I have a right to the information I want." Most of the time this will be true—but it is smart to be expedient about demanding your rights, and not antagonize those with whom you may have to deal amicably later.

Example: A group of residents met regularly in one major city to determine where the power actually rested. Their expectations dwelt initially on highly visible members of the community: the mayor, other politicians, CEOs. However, the group eventually identified a semi-secret business elite who met regularly to discuss the city's politics and business environment and ways to influence them. Though not well known, these parties—professionals and directors of various companies—effectively set the community's agenda. While the discovery was dramatic, classic sleuthing did not bring it about so much as the perseverance and determination of the citizens' group.

Power structure research is a complex matter that is not appropriate for all advocacy efforts. Those who want to explore this area will find further suggestions in "Appendix A," which describes some well-established steps in power structure research, including identifying the relevant information infrastructure, cracking the information bank, and going straight to the source of power for information.

Final words

The process of analyzing root causes—and finding targets for change—carries some traps and limitations that have the potential to throw you off course. For example:

- There's a danger of becoming overwhelmed by the volume of information to be examined. For some, collecting data can become an obsession.
  Suggestion: By monitoring your processes closely, you can ensure that research won't become a substitute for action, or an end in itself. In your group, you should remind yourselves that the point of this step is to understand the problem so you can effectively advocate for change.
- There's a danger of simply becoming overwhelmed by the size of the task facing you.
  Suggestion: If this happens in your group, remind yourselves that not knowing the extent of the problem would be infinitely worse than knowing it—and that it is up to you to select goals for change and targets for change that match your capabilities.

To sum up: "Only believe what you see with your own two eyes—and have your eyes examined regularly." (Collette: *Research Guide for Leaders*) Or: Confirm, reconfirm and (after a while) reconfirm.

"Finding out who is the person behind the name on a deed or board of directors list is essential to understanding what you already know."
BOSTON URBAN STUDY GROUP
WHO RULES BOSTON?

4

Advocacy "Etiquette"

As the saying goes, you don't get a second chance to make a first impression—and the way your health advocacy group approaches an issue can greatly influence your chances of success. Your reputation in the community is one of your most valuable assets, and your actions will affect that reputation both positively and negatively. One early episode of clumsiness or unwanted publicity could throw your entire campaign off track, while a reputation for fairness, toughness and competence can smooth the way throughout the campaign.

We present here twenty guidelines for advocacy "etiquette" compiled from our experience and the experience of other advocates (e.g., Alinsky, 1971; Kahn, 1982). This list is by no means complete, and some guidelines may not be relevant to your situation. However, all of these guidelines have been used by successful advocacy organizations, and they may serve at least as a basis for discussing different approaches for achieving community change. We encourage you to refer back to this chapter as you select your tactics and counter-tactics, many of which employ these principles (see Chapters 7 and 8).

Twenty rules of etiquette

1. Accentuate the positive

Whenever possible, respond to positive events related to your group's mission by thanking others for their actions or paying them public compliments. This is relatively easy, and will differentiate you from the many groups which only speak out when something negative happens. More intrusive or confrontational actions are often best kept for later in a campaign. Having your group perceived as being reasonable (at least some of the time!) will serve it well, if and when you need to take a more confrontational approach.

If you compliment those who support you, acknowledging their wisdom and vision, you are likely to increase their commitment to your goals. For example, a group of citizens concerned about drinking and driving can publicly praise local drinking establishments that have adopted a policy of calling cabs for customers who are drunk. To support this action, they could take out an ad in the local newspaper publicizing the names of these establishments. This low-cost action could very well encourage other establishments to set up a similar policy.

2. Plan for small wins

If there is no evidence of progress, most people can sustain their interest in any issue for only a limited time. Groups are more likely to grow and maintain vitality over time if they experience routine success. One way to achieve this is to develop a plan of action that has steps intermediate to the final goal—and these intermediate victories should be celebrated. Successful efforts will build the confidence and reputation of your group, and make group members more willing to sustain their commitment.

For example, a number of health advocates worked to bring about a small win with McDonalds, the nation's leading fast food chain. Lowering the amount of saturated fat on their menu has been a key objective of many health advocates. One of these, a wealthy businessman and philanthropist, became a nutrition health activist after his personal experience with heart disease. He funded a series of ads criticizing the levels of fat and cholesterol in fast foods, and the appearance of these ads was celebrated by nutrition health advocates. Partly as a result of these ads, McDonalds stopped frying their food in animal fat, began offering low fat and cholesterol alternatives (e.g., low fat muffins, McLean burgers, nonfat milk), and made nutritional information available to consumers. From that beginning, although still not a place where many nutritionists eat lunch, McDonalds has changed enough to become comfortable interacting with public health advocates. At the 1993 annual meeting of the American Public Health Association, for example, McDonalds offered samples of low fat food!

3. Begin by assuming the best of others

When debating your opponents, it may help, at least initially, to assume that their acts are the result of ignorance rather than malice. Challenging the motivations of others can produce needless resistance. If *you* appear suspicious and aggressive, you are likely to generate a similar reaction from your opponent, often leading to a no-win situation. Rather than launching into direct confrontation and criticism, begin with attempts to educate. You may need confrontation later, but it can be counterproductive to adopt this stance in initial efforts.

For example, instead of accusing local or federal agencies of inaction on a health issue, provide them with quality information supporting your position. After all, such agencies are usually underfunded, and have limited resources to maintain effective services or surveillance. If you give them a chance to take action on a given issue, and are disappointed with the results, then you can change your approach—but it is unwise to start fights without giving others the chance to make informed decisions.

In San Jose, California, for example, members of San Jose STAT (Stop Teenage Addiction to Tobacco) were concerned with the number of merchants illegally selling cigarettes to minors. Rather than openly criticizing the code enforcement staff, STAT wrote a detailed proposal to the city advocating a plan for charging merchants a fee that would pay for enforcement of the law. Despite initial resistance, the code enforcement staff presented a report to the city council that was generally positive to the proposed plan. Because San Jose STAT had taken a non-confrontational position, working with, rather than against, city staff, the code enforcement staff did not need to develop strong defensive positions, and were able to appreciate the practical suggestions and help offered by STAT.

4. Do your homework and document your findings

The Scout motto, "Be Prepared," and the statement, "Information is Power" are two pieces of sage advice for the health advocate. It is embarrassing and ineffective to be advocating for an issue on incorrect or incomplete information. The embarrassment of getting the facts wrong can damage a hard-won reputation, direct attention away from the specific issue at hand, and reduce your effectiveness on other issues for which you are advocating, no matter how worthy.

There are many examples of groups whose ability to advocate effectively was compromised because of misinformation. One of the first steps your advocacy group should take is to collect high quality information (see Chapter 3, "Understanding the Issue," for suggestions on documenting the issue) and to become well versed in communicating it (which is discussed in more detail in Chapter 9, "Using the media.") It is important to document the *source* of all information you collect, and to verify it through as many different sources as possible.

Good documentation will strengthen your case, and protect you from denial and counter-charges from the opposition. For example, a consumer group wanting to pass local legislation banning billboards advertising alcohol should compile a list documenting the number and location of billboards, noting which are located near settings where youth congregate (e.g., schools, day care centers, community centers). This will provide evidence for their assertion that billboards are a serious problem.

5. Take the high ground

When you take a position on an issue, try to highlight the general values or principles that relate to your vision—for example, community well-being, health, safe workplaces, a clean community environment, equal access to services, quality of life, and so on. The importance of these values and principles is hard for anyone to deny; thus they serve as a basis for obtaining community consensus. They may also help prevent unresolvable conflicts stemming from disagreements over the details of proposed solutions.

By emphasizing positive values, you will give an air of eloquence to your position that people will find impressive. For example, community well-being, safety, and economic vitality are values usually important to residents faced with the prospect of having a potentially dangerous incinerator located in their community. Keeping these issues in the forefront of discussion can play a key role in the decisions made.

6. Reframe opponents' definitions of the issue

When you are being criticized or attacked by your opponents, try not to respond to the criticism in terms that your opponents have used to define the issue. Rather, reframe it to change the "playing field" (Chapter 7, "Advocacy Tactics," has suggestions on reframing the issue). A key goal is to move support away from your opponent, and toward your group, or the issue for which you are advocating.

The 1992 presidential election presented several examples of this strategy in action. Rather than responding to personal attacks on character or lack of international experience, candidate Clinton kept bringing the debate back to the economy, a topic he had studied intensively and on which the public had strong feelings. Notices reminding workers, "It's the economy, stupid!" were prominently displayed in campaign offices, and Clinton's unwavering attention to that point was a key factor in his election to the presidency.

Another example of turning a negative into a positive occurred in 1965 when Ralph Nader published his book, *Unsafe at any Speed: The Design-in Dangers of the American Automobile.* A private detective was hired by General Motors to find scandal in Nader's life. The detective was caught spying—and when it was revealed that his client was G.M., its president was called before a congressional committee to explain. There he apologized to Nader. The resulting publicity made Nader a folk hero and launched him in his career. Far from damaging him,

G.M.'s attacks diverted attention away from Nader himself, and towards the automobile manufacturers. (This general strategy is discussed in more detail in Chapter 8, "Dealing with the Opposition.")

7. Keep it simple

Sometimes health advocacy groups are drawn to complex actions before giving simpler and easier options a chance. Remember, it is important to have small successes. Focusing only on complex or longer-term strategies may work against your group in this regard. As an example, consider the options of a group of employees who are exposed to hazardous materials without adequate protection. They might consider organizing a strike—but that's a complex action with a high risk of failure. Instead, the group could start with the simple action of filing a grievance with the Occupational Safety and Health Administration (OSHA). If compliance with government regulations does not occur, other more complex and confrontational strategies can then be employed.

8. Be passionate and persistent

On his deathbed, the great scientist, Pavlov, was asked for the secret of success. He said that success depended upon two qualities: passion and persistence. These qualities are especially relevant to health advocacy. If you look at advocacy groups that have been successful, you will find that most have members who are passionate about the issue on which they are advocating, and leaders who live and breathe it. But passion is only part of the equation—and indeed, too much of it can cloud judgment about the choice of appropriate strategies. Persistence, or the unwavering devotion to the cause regardless of obstacles faced, is just as critical to success. Follow-through is a particularly important element of this persistence. If your group establishes a reputation for not following through on commitments or stated intentions, it will be difficult to gain the support of others. Moreover, your opponents will learn to wait until the predictable event occurs—you give up or go away! It's critical that your opponents believe that you will be a burr in their saddle until the issue is resolved.

As community organizer Saul Alinsky noted, "Tactics should maintain a constant pressure upon the opposition. It is this continuous pressure that results in the reactions from the opposition that are essential for the success of a campaign" (Alinsky, 1971). For example, one advocate, Verna Mize, spearheaded efforts to keep the Reserve Mining Company of Minnesota from continuing to pollute Lake Superior in Silver Bay, Minnesota. Her commitment to saving the lake took her through a long process, during which she collected over 25,000 signatures on petitions, recruited the support of many people, filed several civil suits and appeals, picketed, and even provided congressional testimony. She succeeded after seven years of persistence and unwavering passion, even though there were many points where quitting would have been an easier option than fighting on.

9. Be willing to compromise

Developing a healthy community requires cooperation and compromise between groups with competing interests. Although it is important to advocate for your group's cause, you should be open to accepting alternative proposals or compromises that may be advantageous. Being willing to compromise may bring you or your group one step closer to your ultimate goal, engender good feelings and support among key community constituencies, and help improve or sustain your public image.

Public support is almost always on the side of those who are most reasonable in their approach and demands, so compromise is a good strategy provided that it doesn't compromise your group's ultimate goal—the bottom line.

For example, when the city of San Francisco was considering a ban on smoking in public places in late 1993, some tobacco control advocates were keen on including bars in the ban. Realizing that they didn't yet have enough public support for including bars (one of the last bastions of smoking in public places—at least in California), the advocates decided to pull back from the demand. In the end, the ordinance passed in part because advocates had been willing to compromise. However, the fight was not over (remember, passion and persistence are key). Over the next year or two, the advocates planned to rally public and political support for an ordinance addressing the problem of smoking in bars.

10. Be opportunistic and creative

A key skill that health advocates should develop is the ability to wait for the appropriate time for action. That may mean delaying action until you have gathered valid and relevant information; framed the issue in a way that attracts interest and concern; won people's trust in your group; and given people an understanding of the cause for which you are advocating.

Waiting can give you ammunition for your campaign. For example, advocates concerned about the safety of nuclear power plants in their community have waited until the companies refused to disclose safety records. Then the advocates have seized upon this refusal as evidence of mismanagement and lack of good faith. When advocates have publicized these concerns, public trust in the company's sincerity and competence has been compromised. In some cases, this controversy, fueled by negative public sentiment, has discouraged investment in other plants.

"If you are building a house and a nail breaks, do you stop building, or do you change the nail?"
ZIMBABWEAN PROVERB

11. Don't be intimidated

In the process of advocating for health issues, you are likely to encounter opposition from strong individuals or groups. You may choose to avoid confrontation, but it should not be because you are afraid to butt heads with elected officials or corporate executives. Remember that you have access to one powerful weapon: public support. Community health advocates are generally perceived as inherently credible because they are working toward the public good rather than seeking higher profits or social status.

For example, a group of health advocates in Orange County, California approached county health officials with evidence that low income residents were not getting access to health services (Mayster et al., 1990). Addressing this issue involved negotiating with an imposing array of individuals and groups, including local Indigenous Medical Services staff, the Board of Supervisors, the director of the Orange County Health Care Agency, the county administrative officer, the chairman of United Way, the Orange County Medical Association, the Hospital Council of Southern California, and representatives to the state legislature. Had advocates been at all intimidated by working with these powerful individuals and agencies, change might not have occurred.

12. Maintain focus on the issues

Your opponents might try to divert attention from the issue for which you are advocating by attacking group members personally. It is important to avoid falling into that trap. If you take the bait and react to the attacks, confrontation can degenerate into personal animosity, and the group's public image will suffer. For example, groups advocating for increased enforcement and surveillance of drinking and driving laws have been attacked by the beer and alcohol lobby for being anti-business, or supportive of a "police-state." Such name-calling distracts from the issue at hand, and defending yourselves can easily divert your resources away from effective strategies. Keep in mind that, in many cases, your opponents' attempts at discrediting group members are evidence of their inherent vulnerability. While it is tempting to counter accusation with accusation, it is better to avoid being drawn into argument on the issue. Sticking to the high ground and staying focused on the issues at hand is usually more effective in the long run.

13. Make it local and keep it relevant

There's no better way to present an issue than in terms that are close to home. Whenever possible, use local statistics, local role models, and local volunteers in your advocacy efforts. Local issues can mobilize community members concerned

"What keeps you going is that once in a while what you do has an impact on policy, even if it's not exactly what you wanted, even if you get only halfway there."
KARIM AHMED,
NATURAL RESOURCES
DEFENSE COUNCIL

about or directly affected by the issue. Even if your group has support from an organized national campaign, it is *local* support that will ultimately determine your success. In two mid-western states, for example, a group of advocates gathered data on the number of children riding without safety devices, and on public support for requiring that they be used. This information was used to promote adoption of laws in these states regarding the safety of child passengers (Fawcett, Seekins and Jason, 1987).

14. Be broadly based and nonpartisan from the beginning

In many communities, key segments of the health care delivery system, government, and business may initially be suspicious of health advocacy efforts. Nonetheless, health advocacy groups should try to cultivate the cooperation and gain the support of these well-established forces in the community. A commitment to finding reasonable and broadly shared solutions to local health issues is critical to gaining the long-term support and trust of existing organizations. For example, a Wichita, Kansas coalition for the prevention of substance abuse, known as Project Freedom, included representatives from the department of health, human service agencies, businesses, government, religious organizations, schools, law enforcement, and youth and community organizations (Fawcett, Paine, Francisco & Vliet, 1993).

15. Develop an independent public identity

Newly created health advocacy groups should avoid the perception of being "one more program" of a sponsoring organization, or being too closely identified with one of their funders. By tying the advocacy group to the coattails of another group, these perceptions might prove limiting for future projects, and can threaten the credibility of the group. It may take careful planning efforts to develop your own identity, but it is worth the effort, even if you are part of a larger movement. For example, since Ralph Nader suggested in 1970 that students at the University of Oregon create Public Interest Research Groups (PIRGs), students at 140 institutions in some 25 states have organized their own PIRGs. Each one controls its own affairs, hires its own staff, and chooses its own issues and positions. In so doing, each has a unique identify that is easily recognizable.

16. Try to stay within the experiences of individuals in your group

The actions of your group should be consistent with the experience, values, and interests of individual group members. In this regard, it is important to assess group preferences regularly. A typical example is when an advocacy group decides to take an action that might result in members being arrested for trespassing or violating some local ordinance. Some group members may not be ready for such radical action. Group leaders should be careful to avoid this type of situation, which disrupts the group process, and may force some members to leave.

17. Whenever possible, go outside the experience of your opponent

A confused opponent is a weak opponent. Most companies and agencies are not prepared to deal with public opposition to their policies or actions. Likewise, they may not be prepared to deal with unanticipated options dealt to them by advocates. Obviously, going outside the experiences of your opponent requires that you understand your opponents' strengths and weaknesses and how best you can counter them. (See Chapter 8, "Dealing with the Opposition.")

18. Make your opponents live by their own rules

Government and other agencies have explicit policies and regulations that dictate procedures and protocols. When dealing with these agencies, make sure you know those rules, and use them to your benefit. For instance, a consumer group can take advantage of mandatory public hearings to present testimony about the benefits or harms of a given proposal. Citizens can also file appropriate grievances with government agencies responsible for enforcing certain regulations. Once you know all about the agency's procedures and protocols, you may be able to use them to exploit a great many opportunities.

19. Tie advocacy group efforts to related events

Your group should be alert to any event that might be relevant to your objectives or tactics. Linkage to such events can help publicize your cause and strengthen your position. For example, advocates wanting to increase funds and services for patients with a certain disease might publicize a death to draw attention to scarce or unavailable treatment. Similarly, opponents of nuclear power plants can use any reported accident or "near" accident to support their claims.

20. Have a good time

If members of your advocacy group do not take pleasure in their actions, there may be something wrong with your strategy. Saul Alinsky, the legendary community organizer, knew how to make advocacy fun. For example, he once organized a bean feed for his members shortly before they went to a concert also attended by powerful (and dignified) members of the opposition. The result was considerable amusement for the organization's members—something less for their opponents.

If advocacy is fun, lasting ties are more likely to develop among members, along with a growing sense of individual fulfillment and responsibility. A sense of enjoyment, together with a sense of pride, will sustain individual commitment over long periods of time and thus should be nurtured.

Summary

The twenty rules of etiquette presented here will help you to benefit from the experience of thousands of advocacy groups who have gone before you. There is nothing magical about the rules, so they are not recipes for instant success. But they may help bring into focus the philosophical stance that a health advocacy group can take. At a minimum, they should be examined and discussed among group members before action is taken.

5

Making Your Plans

A major challenge for an advocacy organization is to transform the vision and energy of its active members into a strategic action plan. You may not be able to fill in all the details of the plan until you have made decisions about strategic and tactical approaches (see Chapters 6 and 7), but it is important to start on your "road map" now, so that you will have a good sense of direction to guide you through the rest of the process.

This chapter will draw together the work you have done already in developing a vision; and finding and researching an issue. It will guide you through the process of making a mission statement, and setting objectives. It will also help you identify agents of change, targets of change, and settings for change. Finally, it will help you sketch out the broad elements of your campaign. At the end of the chapter, you will find eight worksheets which you may copy and complete as you plan your own campaign. But first, here are some explanations.

Worksheet 1:
Your vision and your mission

Vision

Refer back, if necessary, to the discussion of vision in Chapter 1 as you develop (or polish) your own vision statement. Remember, this statement should be concise and easy to communicate, such as "Drug-Free Streets," "People Power," or "Healthy Babies"—the sort of message that would fit on a T-shirt. If you have not yet verbalized your vision, do so now with the group, and enter it on Worksheet 1 on page 44.

Mission

While your vision refers to your ultimate goal, your mission statement should add information on the what and the why. It is based on your research into the issue, and your analysis of its cause.

A mission statement will act as a guiding star throughout the campaign. It should be quite short and punchy, but give an idea of your role in relation to the vision. For example, if your vision is "Drug-Free Streets," your mission might be "To serve as a catalyst for creating a drug-free community." Alternative mission statements might be, "To find constructive activities for youth"; or, "To eliminate toxic dumping in Murchison County."

You will find the mission statement is frequently useful, serving as a summary of your purpose whenever you talk to community groups, make presentations, or give interviews to the media. Internally, it is helpful in keeping your group focused on its central purpose. For example, before you plan any major strategic or tactical step, you will be able to ask yourselves if this contemplated effort is consistent with your mission. Similarly, when members disagree over strategies and tactics, a reference to the shared mission can help bring the group back together.

When your group has agreed on a mission statement, write it in the space provided on Worksheet 1.

Worksheet 2:
Identifying objectives

Objectives refer to specific, measurable steps that help you reach your goal. Good objectives are SMART: specific; measurable (at least potentially), achievable (at least eventually), relevant (to the mission) and timed (with a date for completion). For example:
- "By the year (x) to reduce cigarette smoking to no more than 15 percent among people in Johnson County."
- "By the year (x) to reduce the estimated pregnancy rate among 12 to 17 year olds in Bay City by 30 percent."
- "By the year (x) to eliminate toxic dumping from Murray County."

The ultimate objective may be months, years or even generations from reality— yet, to survive, movements require victories and the encouragement they provide. Hence, we try to identify intermediate goals that will boost us toward our long-term objective. For example, a cancer-prevention initiative, in addition to the long-term objective of reducing the incidence of cancer, might have such intermediate objectives as these:
- Provide free screening of women identified as high-risk;
- Provide training for lifeguards to encourage reduction in the public's exposure to the sun.

If these intermediate goals themselves might not be readily attainable within a short period of time, a group may establish even shorter-term objectives that boost their power and credibility, and encourage the members. For example, short-term goals related to toxic dumping might include:

- Holding public hearings about the long-term plan for handling toxic waste;
- Forming a committee of physicians and public health officials to provide oversight.

Use Worksheet 2 on page 45 to document short-term, medium-term and long-term objectives. For example:

Long-term objective:
Reduce adolescent pregnancy by 75 percent in Geary County by the year x (four years from now).

Medium-term objective:
Make contraceptives accessible to all high school students by the year x (two years from now).

Short-term objective:
Increase public awareness of the issue of adolescent pregnancy by the year x (one year from now).

Note: your choice of objectives will of course be guided by the extent of your own resources—and those of your allies—in terms of funds, staff and facilities. The research you undertook to document the issue, as described in Chapter 3, will help ensure that your chosen objectives are not out of reach, and that you don't underestimate the strength of the opposition at this point.

Worksheet 3:
Selecting strategies

Strategies are a vital part of the context for action planning. As you will see in the next chapter, strategies refer to how the group intends to do its business. They can include such approaches as advocacy, coalition building, community development, coordination, education, networking, public awareness, and policy or legislative change.

We suggest you read and consider Chapter 6, "Strategy" before you complete the worksheet.

Worksheets 4 and 5:
Choosing targets of change, and agents of change

This part of the planning process may involve referring back to your initial research into the causes and surrounding circumstances of your chosen issue (see Chapter 3).

Through your research, you probably identified certain targets of change (those whose behavior or inaction contributes to the problem) and agents of change (those who are in a position to contribute to the solution).

Examples:
- In a community initiative to control tobacco use by minors, targets of change might include those merchants who sell cigarettes to children;
- In a community effort to reduce risk of injury, agents of change might be parents and teachers who can persuade children to wear bicycle helmets.

Paradoxically, when we consider the list of potential agents or targets of change, we may find some of our most effective "agents" among those who at first sight could be considered "targets." For example, an initiative to address youth violence might draw on the leadership of gang members, or a tobacco control initiative might find an agent of change in a merchant whose knowledge of the business could help advocates devise an approach to other merchants.

Note that the list of targets of change can become quite long, because it will include all those individuals, groups, agencies, businesses or organizations whose behavior needs to change if the mission of the advocacy initiative is to be achieved.

Worksheet 6:
Identifying sectors for change

The more precise you can be in identifying sectors of the community where you want change to take place, the better. Rather than wasting energy by spreading your efforts too wide, you can concentrate on those sectors that are most relevant to your mission, directing your advocacy activities towards them. By keeping your efforts focused, you will avoid the danger of biting off more than you can chew. For an adolescent pregnancy initiative, for example, the best sectors for change might be schools and religious organizations, because these sectors provide access to key targets of change (the youth) and agents of change (peers, parents, teachers, and religious leaders).

The criteria for deciding to involve a community sector are whether (a) it provides access to key targets of change such as youth, merchants or elected officials, and (b) whether it will help you involve key agents of change such as peers, or law-enforcement officials.

Remember not to make your selection of sectors too narrow. Health problems are the result of deficiencies in a variety of environments, and may require changes in multiple sectors, at multiple levels. However, a note of caution is appropriate: although a group's aims must be comprehensive, they should also be focused. While you may have a wide array of aims, you should also set priorities for the sectors where changes are sought, deciding where you should put your energies in each year of the campaign.

Worksheet 6 notes sectors of the community that might be relevant to your advocacy organization, and provides an opportunity for your group to discuss which sectors you will need to target in order to accomplish your mission.

Worksheet 7:
Selecting community changes to be sought

A comprehensive action plan includes an array of changes to be sought in each community sector that is relevant to the organization's mission. A substance abuse coalition, for example, might attempt to bring about a variety of changes in programs, policies and practices in many sectors of the community, including schools, law enforcement, and religious organizations. The challenge now is to decide on a set of changes that will maximize each sector's contribution to the mission.

Here, it is important to avoid a "solution bias" about what changes can be made in each sector, and to keep an open mind. In other words, we should not assume that schools can only provide information; that criminal justice agencies can only enforce laws; that the business community can only provide jobs, and so on. That sort of narrow thinking will limit our ability to maximize each sector's potential contribution to change.

Specific tactics can be filled in at a later date (you will find a list of forty to start with in Chapter 7), but we suggest that here you consider the eight broad categories of tactics that we use in the following example, which shows what changes a substance abuse coalition might seek in each category:

1. **Providing information and skills training**
   Arranging for training of parents and teachers in monitoring for substance abuse.

2. **Providing incentives and disincentives**
   Providing incentives, such as after-hours jobs, for youth who are drug free.

3. **Facilitating support from influential others**
   Establishing peer support groups for youths and parents.

4. **Changing the physical design of the environment**
   Providing adequate night lighting and security on school grounds.

5. **Improving services**
   Developing after-school employment and recreational programs for youth.

6. **Modifying organizational policies**

Establishing a policy of mandatory expulsion from athletics for violating the drug free code.

7. **Providing public information and feedback**

Providing a community scorecard reporting drug and alcohol-related offenses in the community.

8. **Modifying broader public policies**

Changing reporting laws to facilitate public exposure of drug dealers.

Worksheet 8: Preparing action steps

At this point the group should have identified a set of changes that reflect its long- and short-term goals, and its agreed-on priorities. Once the group has achieved this consensus, it is useful to clarify the action steps required to bring about the desired change.

As you consider each action step, ask yourselves the following questions to help you assess the feasibility of the plan, and assign responsibility for its implementation:

- What action needs to be done?
- Who will take that action?
- By what date will that action need to be done?
- What resources and support are needed?
- What resources and support are available?
- What individuals and organizations might resist?

Some groups will not be ready for this step at this time. Consideration of specific actions may need to wait until you have reviewed the possible options available to you, as discussed in the later chapters on the choice of tactics, and the use of media. If that is the case, come back to this chapter later, and complete Worksheet 8, on page 51.

Guiding the process of action planning

The planning process outlined in this chapter may prove to be one that involves hard work, and perhaps high emotions for your group. Frequently, disagreements may lead to discussions of philosophical differences. If these discussions blossom into full-fledged arguments, there is a risk of damaging the unity of the group. Here are six general guidelines to help you cope as amicably as possible with the process of planning outlined in this chapter:

1. **Be inclusive**

   Seek a diversity of viewpoints about what the organization should accomplish.

2. **Manage conflict**

   When conflict occurs among members of the group, try to bring them back to the shared vision and sense of mission, and find common ground.

3. **Use brainstorming rules**

   All members should be able to express ideas without criticism.

4. **Be efficient**

   Negotiate and stick to starting and ending times of meetings.

5. **Communicate products of planning**

   Communicate the results of planning to members and constituents, letting them know when plans are complete.

6. **Provide support and encouragement**

   Let people know who did what and the value it had for the organization.

Completing the plans

As you proceed to complete the worksheets on the following pages, here are two suggestions:
1. Feel free to copy these sheets;
2. Don't feel you need to complete them all at one sitting.

   It may require many meetings, over many weeks or months, before you are satisfied with your plans as a group. For some of the plans, as we said above, you may need more time to explore the options outlined in Chapters 6 through 9.

Worksheet 1

Reviewing your group's vision and mission

Vision

Refer back to Chapter 1 for information on the nature of a vision for advocacy. The vision captures the dream or ideal. It should be very concise, and shared by all.

Examples: Drug-free streets; Clean water; Opportunity for all

YOUR GROUP'S VISION

_____

_____

Mission

The mission statement describes what the advocacy organization needs to do, and why. It should be concise, but expressed in more detail than the Vision.

Examples: "To advocate for a smoke-free Burlington;" "To eliminate toxic waste dumping in Bluff County."

YOUR GROUP'S MISSION:

_____

_____

Worksheet 2

Identifying objectives

Refer to page 38 for help on developing objectives. To remind you, they should be SMART: Specific, measurable (at least potentially), achievable (at least eventually), relevant (to the mission) and timed (including a date for completion). They should answer the questions, "What? Who? Where? By how much? And by when?" Some advocacy campaigns may have several objectives: others may be focused on one or two.

Example: By the year x, to reduce the number of children and youth who start using tobacco in Monroe County by 50 percent.

LONG TERM OBJECTIVES

1. _____

   _____

2. _____

   _____

MEDIUM TERM OBJECTIVES

1. _____

   _____

2. _____

   _____

SHORT TERM OBJECTIVES

1. _____

   _____

2. _____

   _____

Worksheet 3

Selecting strategies

See Chapter 6 for information about selection of strategies. A strategy should provide the broad road by which you will reach your objectives—for example through coalition building; educational approaches; policy change, and so on. Remember that multiple approaches are generally more effective than one single approach.

Example: "Increase awareness of dumping through public demonstrations."

YOUR GROUP'S STRATEGIES:

1. _____

_____

_____

_____

2. _____

_____

_____

_____

3. _____

_____

_____

_____

4. _____

_____

_____

_____

Worksheet 4

Choosing targets of change

Targets of change include all those who need to change, either because they are at risk (i.e. adolescents, children, pregnant mothers) or because a change in their behavior would reduce the risk to others (merchants, government agencies, service providers, etc.)

YOUR GROUP'S TARGETS OF CHANGE

1. _____

_____

2. _____

_____

3. _____

_____

4. _____

_____

5. _____

_____

6. _____

_____

7. _____

_____

8. _____

_____

Worksheet 5

Choosing agents of change

Agents of change are those who are in the best position to contribute to a solution. They might be peers; parents; caregivers; service providers; business people; elected officials, etc.

AGENTS OF CHANGE RELEVANT TO YOUR GROUP'S OBJECTIVES

1. _____

2. _____

3. _____

4. _____

5. _____

6. _____

7. _____

8. _____

Worksheet 6

Identifying sectors for change

Below is a diagram of community sectors that might be targeted by your advocacy organization. Ask yourselves which community sectors should be used to address your group's mission? Which of these offer good prospects for changing the behavior of your "targets of change"? Which might be valuable in reaching and involving your potential "agents of change"?

On this diagram, mark those sectors that will be addressed by your advocacy organization (and add additional sectors, if the ones you plan to involve are not represented.)

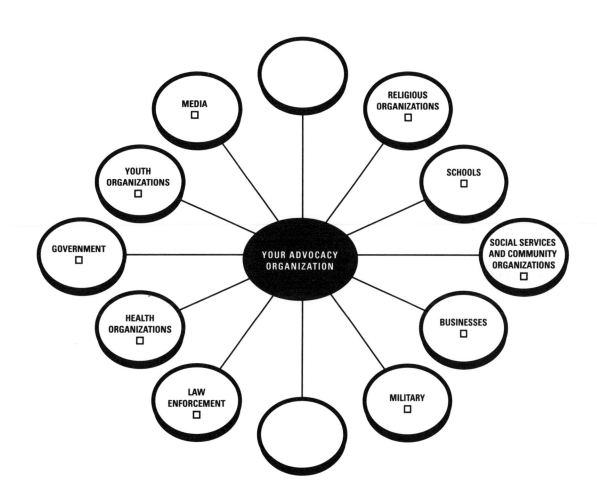

Worksheet 7

Selecting community changes to be sought

Use this planning page to identify the specific community changes to be sought in each sector. Indicate your plans in each of the eight areas of action identified on pages 41-42. Use the examples given on those pages as your guide. Copy this page, and use one worksheet for the changes you plan in each community sector.

COMMUNITY SECTOR: _____

Providing information and skills training: _____

_____

Providing incentives and disincentives: _____

_____

Facilitating support from influential others: _____

_____

Changing the physical design of the environment: _____

_____

Improving services: _____

_____

Modifying policies of related organizations: _____

_____

Providing public information and feedback: _____

_____

Modifying broader public policies: _____

_____

Worksheet 8

Selecting action steps

Make a copy of this sheet for each of the community sectors where you will seek changes. Provide information in the categories described on page 42.

COMMUNITY SECTOR: _____   **CHANGE TO BE SOUGHT:** _____

Action	By whom	By when	Resources & support needed / available	Organizations or people who might resist

6

Strategy

Once you know where you want to go, the question is, how can you get there? Realistically, *how* can you:

- Break down bureaucratic resistance?
- Have influence over decision-makers?
- Effect real change?

Even if the kitchen table is national headquarters, a small group is a force to be reckoned with if it believes in what it is doing, keeps on doing it with passion and persistence, and has a good strategy. These strategies, which will be the key to your success, should be in place well before action is taken. Unfortunately, some advocates jump to action without thinking about the strategic context within which that action is taken. This can lead to false starts and ineffective advocacy.

In the next chapter, we will discuss the tactics that will enable you to carry out your strategy. In this chapter, we will give you suggestions for thinking about different strategic styles, with references to the research that might help you select an appropriate strategy.

What is strategy?

Strategy refers to *how* the group intends to do its business. It can include such approaches as advocacy, coalition building, community development, coordination, education, networking, public awareness, and policy or legislative change.

Here is one way of looking at the terminology of a campaign:

- Your group has the *mission* of providing shelter.
- You fix an *objective*: you plan to build a house.
- The architectural design and blueprints constitute your *strategy*.

- The methods used in the cement, carpentry, plumbing and electrical work will be your *tactics*.
- Providing the tools and materials, and scheduling the workers constitutes your *action plan*.

One way that advocates may get bogged down is by failing to distinguish between strategies and tactics, or by getting enamored of certain tactics. As Bobo et al. noted in *Organizing for Social Change:*

> All too often, organizations allow a tactic to take on a life of its own, independent of any strategic context. When this happens, a group will hear of a clever tactic that worked someplace else, and use it without considering why it worked the first time, or how their situation might be different...The worst mistake an organizer can make is to act tactically instead of strategically.

The traditional military distinction between strategy and tactics is also useful: *Strategy* provides your broad plan, and the approach for achieving your objective; *Tactics* are your actions for carrying out strategy.

Sample strategies

Here is a brief list of sample strategies—in this case for a campaign to reduce sales of tobacco to minors. Notice that they don't spell out the way that actions are to be taken:

- Increasing public awareness
- Skill building for prevention/cessation
- Education of merchants
- Modifying access to tobacco
- Surveillance
- Enforcement
- Increasing cost of behavior
- Policy change
- Coordination and networking

A list of tactics would include much more specific actions, such as "set up a sting," "hold a press conference," or "send an educational mailing to merchants."

Strategic styles

In addition to deciding about what practical form your strategy will take, and what you will do, you will also need to decide how you will carry it out. For example—to continue the military analogy—different strategic styles might include the following:

- To conduct an all-out assault with guns blazing;
- To infiltrate your spies into the enemy camp;
- To work on the population through propaganda and persuasion;
- To ask for a summit meeting with the opponent;
- To build slowly on small victories.

Strategic approaches can cover a broad range of styles, from "social action" to "social planning." At one extreme is the intrusive, in-your-face street demonstration, like those by ACT UP or similar activists. At the other extreme, you would find the gentle, research-based persuasiveness of groups like the League of Women Voters. For many, the most effective approach might lie somewhere in between. What is important, however, is to recognize that communities change, circumstances change, and the way that different segments of the community are connected to each other may be in a constant state of flux. The strategy you start with will not necessarily be the best one to finish with.

Recognizing connections and change

One strategic approach, called "systems advocacy," involves paying careful attention to the way that different parts of the community are related to each other. It's not "us" and "them"—we are all in this together. Most segments of a community, such as public health, safety, education and recreation, share common interests. These groups are all connected to each other in an informal network that attempts to serve the interests of the community as a whole.

Systems advocacy begins with that idea of connection. It recognizes that we are all linked, and our actions, whether individually or in groups, affect others. Even citizens acting individually have some influence on the beliefs, attitudes, and actions of neighbors. We all participate in one way or the other in community structures and systems, which influence each of us.

People generally act in their own interests, but they change with time, and so do their interests. Change in interests can occur when we gain a new insight — perhaps as a result of personal experience, or the influence of family, friends, colleagues, mentors, employers or others. The view of a person who strenuously objects to government restrictions of smokers' rights, for example, might be moderated upon hearing that his children's twelve-year-old friends are smoking.

This is how interests evolve in public policy debates. Views are not set in granite, for the most part, but are frequently challenged. Informed citizens express concerns to neighbors, organizations and elected representatives. Organizations raise issues with the public and decision-makers. The media report on issues, and give different perspectives about them. Policy-makers look for areas where people are most likely to agree.

It may be helpful in considering your own community to see how individual community members and groups negotiate and benefit from one another, in order for all of them to increase their effectiveness. Keep in mind:

1. People are more likely to choose a course of action if there is some sign or direct evidence that it will be to their benefit—and vice versa. They are likely to avoid action when it might bring pain or punishment.
2. People will tend to pursue those activities and associations they find rewarding and fair, and avoid those they do not.
3. Benefits must be sustained, and strategies should be evaluated at regular intervals to see whether people are getting what they need and desire. (see Chapter 10, "Evaluating Health Advocacy Organizations.")

Choosing strategies

Any strategy has limitations that may leave you short of your objective. Each situation has its own players, interests, history and conditions. It is important to choose a strategy that fits the particular circumstances. Take the example of a nursing home which provides inadequate care:

- The hammer of an "in-your-face" social action strategy, such as a boycott or picketing, will be counterproductive for reforming the home if the kindly, sweet operator is doing her best under severe state budget restraints.
- A social planning strategy, such as the collection and presentation of facts at the local level, may offer little when we know that the real source of the problem is some committee in the state legislature.
- A strategy encouraging individuals and groups to solve their own problems would also have limitations in this hypothetical instance, since the affected family members and residents of the home probably lack the resources to make up the deficiencies themselves.

About direct action

Should you adopt a strategy of nonviolent direct action, which might include sit-ins, or blocking traffic? You will find more on this in Chapter 8, "Dealing with the Opposition." Nonviolent direct action has been shown to enhance group unity, morale and solidarity in the face of oppression, but it should not be used lightly—and usually only when less confrontational methods have been tried and have failed.

Matching issues and strategies

Here is one method of selecting a strategic direction according to the situation. It assumes there are four types of community situations that might affect the strategic direction you take: good news; rumors; unmet needs; bad news. There are four strategic goals which are generally appropriate responses to these situations. Put them together and you have the makings of a campaign.

SITUATION	STRATEGIC GOAL
Good news	Reinforce
Rumors	Investigate, correct
Unmet needs	Reverse, correct
Bad news	Reverse, correct

"A roaring lion kills no game."

Tanzanian proverb

Good news

This type of situation occurs when actions by others are compatible with your group's values, goals and plans—for example, when others make positive changes in policies, regulations, services, or proposals. If you are a coalition whose aim is to combat heart disease, and a local grocery chain says it will be emphasizing healthy food choices, that's good news. It's consistent with your objective of increasing the availability of products that are beneficial to health. Generally, the appropriate strategy is to reinforce the actions that contribute to your objective. (For specific tactics, see Chapter 7.)

Rumors

Another common situation is the circulation of unsubstantiated claims about the plans or motivations of others. For example, a member of your group may hear that the school board plans to stop making contraceptives available through school clinics, which will endanger your objective of reducing teenage pregnancy. The appropriate response, or strategy, is an investigation to determine whether this is true. Tactics for carrying out that strategy might include tracing the rumor to its point of origin, or reviewing recent minutes of school board meetings.

Unmet needs

It may be that your research into the needs of your community (see Chapter 3) revealed that major problems facing people are simply not being addressed effectively. The appropriate strategy here may be to create options to fill the need—whether by bringing about improvement in existing programs, or putting pressure on the agencies responsible for establishing new ones.

Bad news

In this type of situation, others take action that is contrary to your values, goals and plans. Faced with negative proposals, or changes in policies, regulations or services, your strategy is to prevent implementation or to force change. It may be especially important to make a quick response, to ensure that the policy-makers won't underestimate the significance of the damaging development.

Summary:
Tactics and strategies, means and not ends

Many people select weapons, strategies or tactics with which they personally feel comfortable, rather than ones which would be most effective based on an analysis of what is really needed. Some people try to organize a demonstration to deal with every issue because they 'love' demonstrations. Others have a strong belief in 'getting everyone together to talk about it,' and they follow that approach whether it is effective or not in a particular instance. If you are really interested in impact as well as the fun of the process, you have to analyze the nature of the problem before prescribing a remedy.
—Bobo et al.

The take-home point here is to allocate substantial time to developing your strategy. Shortcutting this step in the advocacy process is certain to reduce your effectiveness. Refine your strategy numerous times, and test it out with trusted friends and colleagues. Then, when you are confident about it, stick to it.

An excellent resource for helping you develop a strategy, and linking it to tactics, is *Organizing for Social Change: A Manual for Activists in the 1990s,* by Kim Bobo, Jackie Kendall and Steve Max (see "References" on page 159). It offers the "Midwest Academy Strategy Chart," which can help you develop a comprehensive strategy and tie it into a campaign. The chart includes goals; organizational considerations; constituents, allies, and opponents; targets; and tactics.

7

Advocacy Tactics

"Consider how hard it is to change yourself and you'll understand what little chance you have of trying to change others."

JACOB M. BRAUDE

Once your group has outlined a campaign plan, and you have an idea of the strategy you will follow, it is time to start giving tactical form to the campaign. In this chapter, you will find some general principles to guide your actions, and suggestions for the different types of tactics you can use. Although some of the tactics we suggest may seem like "quick fixes," remember that the campaign itself may be a long one: social change usually takes time, as issues may need to "marinate" in the social fabric before they lead to actual change.

Campaigns will take shape differently, depending on the circumstances and the issue. Usually, you can't expect to plan every detail up front. After the initial actions your choice of tactics may be dictated by the reaction of others, and adjusted in response to external forces over which the group has no control. (See Chapter 8, "Dealing with the Opposition.")

Here are some reminders from earlier sections of the book:

- You will need a strong factual base for your position, based on thorough knowledge of the issue;
- You may need a broad base of community support from which to operate, perhaps provided by a coalition of like-minded organizations;
- You will need to know about available resources, including funds and volunteers;
- You will need high group morale, with a shared sense of purpose.

Six principles

Here is a list of six principles that, if adopted as policy, will enhance your tactical efforts:

Presence

Once engaged in an issue, do something about it frequently. Because you are attempting to shape the behavior of others, their consciousness about the issue is crucial, so you should make sure that they are reminded of the issue regularly.

Generosity

Be generous in your praise of others for their strengths and actions. Generous groups are viewed positively by the public, and this good will is an important asset. Praise also increases the likelihood that others will continue to do good things.

Shaping

Reward those who move even a little way towards your goals, because achieving community change is like shaping clay. You can't do it all at once.

Escalation

If the first efforts are not successful, expand your efforts for subsequent actions. Overcome resistance by mobilizing greater numbers of proponents, increasing the effort you put into tactics, and showing greater intensity in the way you articulate feelings about the issues.

Accuracy and honesty

Be scrupulously accurate in all written or spoken statements represented as fact, denying opponents any opportunity to prove you are wrong. Your credibility and, more important, the issue itself are on the line.

Consistency

If you praise or criticize one group for a particular position, treat others the same.

"We did not decide whether or not an action would succeed; we were unconcerned about whether or not a position was popular. What was important was the doing, the process, organic in that it expands, takes root, grows shoots or even dies."

POLLY MANN,
PEACE CALENDAR

Making choices

Each campaign has a style and personality of its own because it is a composite of the group and its actions, and each choice should reflect that tone. Bear that in mind as you answer questions like these:

- Will a militant, confrontational approach be consistent with your image, and with the sentiments of the public or decision-makers who are in the position to force change?
- If your opening shot is an extreme one—such as a boycott—what tactics will be left if that fails and it becomes necessary to escalate?
- Does it make sense to discuss forming a community conference on an issue when all evidence indicates there is inadequate interest?

The great number of choices can be overwhelming, but as health advocates you are not starting from scratch. This chapter presents specific tools that others have used in their own advocacy campaigns. Some of these tactics may work for you; some won't. At all times, remember that the tactics offer only a starting point. Your group can be as creative as it likes in combining tactics, or inventing new ones.

Framing the issue

As you will see from many of the tactics presented here. One of the most basic requirements for a successful campaign is to frame the issue on your own terms, not on those used by the opposition. All members of the organization who have contact with the press, the public or the opposition should be constantly aware of the need to put the group's own spin on the issue.

Here is an example of the different ways that an advocacy group and its opponents might frame an issue—in this case, concerning tobacco use. Tobacco industry framing is given first, with pro-advocacy framing following in bold:

- Smoking is a matter of personal choice;
  People smoke because they are addicted.
- Smoking bans discriminate against smokers;
  Non-smokers have the right to breathe clean air.
- Smoking bans infringe on personal freedom;
  Smoking bans protect public health.
- The tobacco companies do good through sponsorship of cultural, athletic and community events;
  The tobacco companies attempt to gain innocence by association.
- We don't need more government regulation—just common sense, courtesy and accommodation;
  Voluntary approaches don't work.

"Finding the energy to sustain activism long enough to become skilled at it, long enough to make a real difference in this impervious, consuming society—to be able to avoid burn-out and yet not simply go through the motions—is an art."
PAT FARREN,
PEACE CALENDAR

- Smoking bans are public health fascism;
  Smoking bans are public health protection.
- Tobacco is just one of many presumed health hazards.
  Why don't we regulate fat?
  Tobacco is the only legal product that when used as intended, kills.

(For a vivid demonstration of framing the issue in a presentation, see Appendix B.)

Categorizing advocacy tactics

It is helpful when considering tactics to divide them up according to your purpose, and the different stages of the campaign. We have divided the forty tactics presented here into three broad categories:

1. **Tactics for Research and Investigation**

2. **Tactics for Encouragement and Education**

3. **Direct Action Tactics**, which are further subdivided into four sections:
   - Making your presence felt
   - Mobilizing public support
   - Using the system
   - Getting serious.

The categories as presented here offer a natural sequence, starting with a firm basis of research. They don't progress to direct action without attention to education of both the public and, if appropriate, the opposition. Within each group, tactics generally escalate from the less intrusive to the more intrusive.

We suggest that advocates consider a wide range of possible tactics within each category at this point, remembering that it is usually advisable to bring to bear as many advocacy tactics as you can, provided that you have the capacity to carry them out, and they fit your mission, strategy and context. However:

- Don't think you have to do everything; consider only those tactics that directly address the strategy selected.
- Don't think you need to follow the order in which tactics are presented here; each community will have to decide when to do what.
- Use these tactics as a starting point; be creative in your use of combinations of existing tactics, or your invention of new ones. Some may strike you as essential, others irrelevant. As always, the choice about which actions to employ belongs, ultimately, to the group.

Tips

Here's one final list of tips before you reach our list of tactics. These were taken from Cliff Douglas and Jack Claypoole (1992), who developed a set of concrete suggestions for those involved in tobacco control ad vocacy, including these:

- Be knowledgeable of the "game" in which you are playing. As with all games, being "right" does not guarantee winning.
- Be knowledgeable of the position about which you are advocating; stay focused on it, and share it with your allies.
- Be careful to distinguish between working hard and working smart.
- Start your efforts early, and have backup plans in case your initial strategy fails.
- Be able to mobilize a network of influential advocates to make phone calls, write letters, or meet with decision-makers on short notice.

Tactics for research and investigation

1. Conduct studies of the issue
2. Gather data on public opinion
3. Study the opposition
4. Request accountability
5. Demonstrate commercial benefits
6. Document complaints
7. Act as a watchdog
8. Organize consumer service audits

These tactics provide information to advocates. They go beyond the broad research that contributes to our understanding of the problem (as outlined in Chapter 3), and involve the collection of specific facts that can be used tactically.

1. Conduct studies of the issue

Understanding the issue as fully as possible is the logical starting point. If you have only a surface knowledge of it, this it will limit your ability to identify options and potential allies.

Without specific knowledge, you may not be able to present your arguments as forcefully as you would like. For example, for a campaign with the mission of reducing alcohol use by minors, do you know the true extent of alcohol sales to kids in your community? How knowledgeable are local police about the problem? Are merchants aware of the laws regulating sales to minors? Do you have up-to-date and accurate facts about the alcohol industry, trade groups, distributors and the effects of alcohol on youth? A study committee is essential. Three or more volunteers may suffice, although if the issue is very complex you may require outside help, or help from allied groups.

Potential benefits
This tactic increases understanding of the issue; contributes to the group's resolve; empowers group members by getting them involved in a vital task; and enhances the group's credibility.

2. Gather data on public opinion

If you have access to existing data, or the resources to commission your own surveys, evidence of public concern about health issues can be invaluable. For example, advocates used research data on constituents' willingness to support the laws when they pressed for passage of child passenger safety legislation in Kansas and Illinois (Fawcett, Seekins and Jason, 1987).

If you cannot find existing sources of useful data, it can be gathered by trained volunteers—for example, in surveys of shoppers at a mall. Focus groups, in which eight to twelve people discuss issues under the guidance of a moderator, can produce in-depth reactions that can be informative. Communicating the findings of polls and focus groups to elected officials and other community decision-makers will encourage them to keep health issues on their agenda. Data can provide a basis for press releases (see Chapter 9 for more on using the media). And, of course, data can inform your own tactical decisions throughout the campaign.

Potential benefits
Information is power. The more information you have, the more effective you will be, if you can make use of it. Gathering and disseminating public opinion data can move even the most stubborn opponents.

3. Study the opposition

For any but the most quick-hit campaigns, it can be helpful to establish and maintain contact with the opposition, whether it's the Chamber of Commerce or the local restaurant association, a government agency or a school board, a local hospital or a factory that's polluting the air. For example, maintaining communication with a restaurant association that opposes stricter measures to protect nonsmokers will keep you abreast of its positions, and help you develop effective counter-arguments. By maintaining contact, you may be able to influence policy or practices. You may also be able to head off major confrontations before they flower into a public controversy that could make it harder to reach agreement at a later stage.

Potential benefits

Information on the opposition, especially its strategy and tactics, can help your group evaluate the appropriateness of your own strategies and tactics.

4. Request accountability

Formally asking a responsible party, by letter, for the reasons behind a decision or action may give you a rationale previously unknown to you or others. For example, if local government agencies are definitely failing to enforce existing laws regulating disposal of hazardous waste, write to a responsible party asking for the reasons behind their action (or inaction). Send copies to key decision-makers to alert them of your inquiry. Your request may lead to additional action if the response is unsatisfactory, or is ignored.

The down side may be that by laying your own cards on the table, you alert the opposition to your presence, and may encourage it to mobilize its defenses early.

Potential benefits

Such monitoring can force decision-makers to be more aware of the consequences of their decisions, and the standards they use for reaching them. You may also gather information for use in further actions, formal and otherwise—or even discover new issues.

5. Demonstrate commercial benefits

In this tactic, groups of consumers systematically review the effect of control efforts in the commercial sector, and provide feedback to businesses that are in competition with each other. For example, you could collect data to show that the community supports those stores that refuse to sell tobacco to minors. These data would prove convincing to stores whose policy on the matter is lax.

Potential benefits

Documenting the true extent of financial impact, and not just anecdotal opinions, can persuade even your staunchest critics to re-evaluate their position. Presenting your group as a valid source of information can increase trust in you, and can result in future benefits and power.

6. Document complaints

A group must be extremely careful not to act on complaints that turn out to be based on false premises. Launching a major campaign against a factory that has been accused of polluting ground water is inadvisable if that factory has cleaned up its act, and another is at fault. The resulting embarrassment could be costly, or even

> "I think the most important thing to do is to understand what your power is and how to be able to use limited resources most effectively."
> AN ADVOCATE

fatal, to your purpose. Before acting on any complaint, members of your group should collect relevant documents, and interview witnesses or people with complaints. You should also maintain complete files of the evidence gathered.

Potential benefits
Documenting evidence protects the group from later denials—and documenting complaints sometimes resolves the problem.

7. Act as a watchdog

This involves attending meetings of target organizations when they schedule discussions of interest to you. To do this, you need schedules, so that one or more volunteers can attend and observe meetings quietly (remembering that your presence may arouse suspicion).

Potential benefits
You will gain more information, and perhaps make contacts that will be useful to your group.

8. Organize consumer service audits

In this tactic, groups of consumers systematically compare the quality and usefulness of services from different agencies, and provide positive and corrective feedback to providers. Such comparisons can often pressure competing groups into improving services. On the down side, there may be resentment from agencies not faring so well in the audits. Providers may even refuse service to members, knowing they are acting as monitors.

Potential benefits
There may be improvement of services, while your group gains visibility; goodwill from those receiving positive feedback; an improved base in consumer affairs; and information that may be shared with other consumers.

Tactics for encouragement and education

9. Give personal compliments and public support
10. Arrange celebrations
11. Develop proposals
12. Establish contact and request participation
13. Prepare fact sheets

14. Offer public education
15. Provide corrective feedback

Tactics for encouragement and education help define the terms of debate, and provide support for (or opposition to) people who are joined in that debate.

9. Give personal compliments and public support

Little more is involved than thanking an individual or group for an action you support with a telephone call or letter. You want to reinforce the action and encourage similar activities. Recognizing people who have helped your cause can go a long way in building support for future endeavors (though be careful not to hurt the feelings of potentially important allies by leaving them out). You can spread your praise further by writing letters to the local newspaper editor, or to appropriate public officials.

Potential benefits

You will benefit from: visibility for the group and good public relations; increased probability that the action will continue, and that similar future action will occur; public education about the issue; and increased chances that your group will be involved in future decision-making. In addition, this tactic can lay the groundwork for future coalition-building.

10. Arrange celebrations

How do you recharge dedicated members and volunteers, or recognize project supporters? Having a light side helps. Depressing though your issue may be at times, your prospects for success will be limited if your prevailing mood is somber and workaholic. Those in the trenches for the cause need recognition and a release valve. Partying once in a while is one readily available tool. Resources are simple—a reason to celebrate, a place, a few bucks, some volunteers to pull it together, and the group's willingness and energy for fun. One word of warning: if you are holding a party to honor someone, make sure before you commit yourself that there will be sufficient interest. It can be embarrassing if only a handful of people show up.

Potential benefits

You will have an opportunity to recognize meritorious service or action, and give fun to group members. Your celebration may be of interest to local media. It also provides a chance for release of tension; boosts morale; demonstrates and cements the bond among members; humanizes the group and its objective; and acknowledges outstanding efforts, both inside and outside the group.

11. Develop a proposal

This involves preparing a detailed plan to show how you think a problem should be addressed. Your plan will need to include information about the resources needed for implementation, and the individuals or agencies that would be responsible. It will have to be practicable. The weight and attention given to such an effort will depend in large part on how well the proposal was pulled together, and on the credentials of those responsible for it. You can improve the chances of having a positive effect by producing a well-documented study to back up your proposed plan, and by getting other organizations to collaborate on it (provided that their presence doesn't dilute your objectives).

Potential benefits
Developing a proposal can increase the group's visibility; focus attention on a proposed solution to the problem; give opportunities for group members to participate in a project that could give them valuable experience; and help group members make new contacts.

12. Establish contact and request participation

In Tactic No. 3 under "Research and Investigation," we recommended studying the opposition. For this tactic, you can move in a little closer, and even participate in the opposition's decision-making processes. You may even get into a position to influence policy or practices, or at least to resolve disagreements quietly, avoiding the complications that frequently flow from public controversy. The opposing agency's cooperation can make the process easier (and can help reduce tension) but it is frequently unnecessary, since many board meetings are open. Sometimes an exchange of newsletters or minutes of board meetings is sufficient, though it is more useful to seek participation in an organization's planning sessions. For this, someone will need to make the request, and one or more members knowledgeable about the topic, or willing to learn, must be ready to attend various meetings. In the event a request for participation is denied—and this may happen—it may be necessary to escalate action.

Potential benefits
You may gain valuable experience and contacts; have the chance to influence the target organization's decisions; enhance your group's respectability and credibility; and develop a working relationship with staff in the target organization.

13. Prepare fact sheets

You may find it helpful to have a committee of group members develop two sheets: one about your group, the other about the issue. This will encourage you to develop clear statements about your group's objectives, and about relevant aspects of the issue. Such sheets serve many purposes. They can be included in press packets (see Chapter 9) and handed out whenever members of your organization interface with the public.

Potential benefits

Fact sheets provide readily available resources for media and other inquiries. They help group members maintain consistency and continuity in the message you give to the world.

14. Offer public education

This step is appropriate when your issue (or your group) becomes too big for simple fact sheets and responses to periodic telephone queries. It is useful to entrust some volunteers with the job of organizing an ongoing public information program—supplying material to radio, television, newspapers and newsletters; answering questions; and addressing decision-makers and community groups. (More on these topics in Chapter 9.) A systematic approach to "going public" will help you to make a wider audience aware of the group's purpose, and will ensure that the messages people hear about you and your issue are consistent.

Potential benefits

You will gain public awareness of your group and its issue; opportunities for the group to gain exposure in public settings; and opportunities to develop experience and contacts.

15. Provide corrective feedback

An attack on your group can present an opportunity to explain your point of view, and offer suggestions for corrective steps. In some cases, this will mean writing a letter, or personally contacting those responsible for the offensive words or actions. In other cases, you may reply by way of the media—though it may be wise to avoid embarrassing the target, and inviting retaliation.

Potential benefits

This tactic will give you an opportunity to join the debate on your terms. You can teach the opposition about your group and your issues, or put the record straight so that they use appropriate terms when they represent you in future.

Direct action tactics: Making your presence felt

16. Postpone action
17. Establish an alternative system or program
18. Establish lines of communication with the opponent's traditional allies
19. Criticize unfavorable actions
20. Express opposition publicly
21. Remind those responsible
22. Make a complaint
23. Lobby decision-makers

"Making your presence felt" can involve both positive and negative actions (or in the case of the first of these tactics, taking no action at all).

16. Postpone action

Once you have identified and researched your issue, it's tempting to go public—but often the best tactic at this point is to postpone action. Although too much postponement can mean paralysis, letting issues "marinate" for a limited time may lead to more effective actions later on. For example, if you show your hand too early, you may give targets a chance to cover up, while many facts are yet to be determined.

Is there a downside to postponing action? Yes, if the situation might get worse if you don't act, or people get used to it. In some cases, silence at this stage might be viewed as acceptance, or tacit agreement. Or postponing action might simply be an excuse for procrastination. On the other hand, postponing action becomes a positive tactic when it is backed up by continuous monitoring in anticipation of further action—for example, if you decide not to criticize a city council member for opposing a ban on alcohol billboards near schools until you have a chance to talk, face to face. Or you may have a stronger case for boycotting a store that sells tobacco to minors if you first give the manager a reasonable chance to change his practices.

Potential benefits
This tactic will demonstrate your patience and restraint—and help you avoid rash or unnecessary actions.

17. Establish an alternative system or program

If things are not working well, try something different. Provide a service where there is none, or offer better alternatives to what does exist. In some cases, if you have the people, the funds, the facilities and the expertise, this might mean implementing a program yourselves—i.e., providing activities for youth, or nutrition education, or parenting classes. In other cases, it might mean finding out whether some other agency can take up the slack. For example, if law enforcement agencies are unwilling to enforce laws regulating public drunkenness, determine whether local government agencies with code enforcement responsibility can be used for this purpose. Or talk the school board into providing additional training for youth.

Potential benefits

This tactic can give you control of the program; visibility for your group and the issue; and the satisfaction of knowing that things are getting done.

18. Establish lines of communication with the opponent's traditional allies

You can exploit differences that exist within and between industries, corporations or organizations—a tactic that could be called "dividing the elite." Where business or industry are involved, an advocate group might make a formal alliance with business partners (see Robert N. Mayer's *The Consumer Movement* for examples of such consumer-business coalitions). In other cases, independent lobbying efforts by the advocate group and by business interests simply reinforce each other, even when they are not acting together.

Many of these alliances can be found in the auto industry. Consumer groups link up with manufacturers of fuel-efficient cars against manufacturers of cars with lower fuel efficiencies in the quest for higher fuel-efficiency standards. Or insurance companies may work with consumer groups to establish industry standards for automatic seat restraint requirements. The challenge is to gain leverage without being co-opted by the business community. Some consumer activists feel that if the effort means forfeiting their own objectives, or losing their natural allies, the tactic is not worth it.

Potential benefit

This offers a way to put pressure on the target organization. It can also help you gain resources, and have access to expertise.

19. Criticize unfavorable action

Responding to some unfavorable decision or action, you personally contact or write a letter to those responsible, or to the media, and offer suggestions about possible corrective action. The intent is to modify the action, and decrease the chances that it will happen again—preferably without antagonizing powerful opponents. For example, if your campaign involves tobacco use, you might identify cases where politicians are known to be accepting industry contributions. Or you might find that local stores are displaying an excessively large number of tobacco promotions. Your first step should be to contact those responsible, offering suggestions for possible corrective action. If you don't get a response, then you can escalate to further action—for example, by taking out an advertisement in the paper revealing the extent of the tobacco industry contributions.

Potential benefits:
In addition to changing the situation, you may sensitize the target group to the issue; increase credibility for your group; and mobilize public opinion around your perspective.

20. Express opposition publicly

This tactic involves stating your opposition to some proposal or action through letters to decision-makers; letters to newspapers; testimony at public hearings; or statements at a news conference. The objective is to correct what has occurred, or thwart some objectionable proposal from being implemented. Preparations for a news conference ideally begin at least three weeks in advance, although they can be mounted faster if necessary. (See Chapter 9 for more information on organizing news conferences, and on preparing your spokespeople to state your case.) Take care not to get your group branded as too negative, which may reduce your effectiveness in the long run.

Potential benefits:
In addition to correcting a situation, your group will gain visibility, help educate the public, and increase the chances of being consulted in the future.

21. Remind those responsible

When individuals or organizations fail in their duty, fail to respond to proposed solutions, or fail to follow through on a promise in a timely fashion, remind them of their obligation—mentioning the original promise, and the deadline for action, if there was one. For example, remind an elected official of a campaign promise he or she made on gun control. Or remind a billboard company of its commitment to donate free space for pro-health messages. This tactic should increase the chance that the target will take appropriate action, or at least it might elicit a formal response.

In some cases, you may find that unforeseen problems have developed since the commitment was made. If that is the case, your group might be able to help remove those obstacles. If you receive a negative response, then it might be appropriate to escalate the action.

Potential benefits
This tactic gives the target the benefit of the doubt, and your group a reputation for reasonableness. Your reminder may be genuinely helpful if the target has forgotten the commitment.

22. Make a complaint

Before you file a formal complaint (see Tactic 30), try one that is less formal. Contact the organization or individual responsible for an action directly, making clear the reasons for your objections. (Does an action of theirs violate some agreement, policy or law? Is it harmful to the population at large, or to isolated groups?) The objective is to rectify some improper action without public conflict, and without jeopardizing or embarrassing individuals. Your initial approach should be simply to set forth changes you would like to see, and the reasons behind your proposals. If the target denies the facts you present, you can turn the situation to your advantage, and take this opportunity to clarify the issue.

Potential benefits

This tactic may help to head off public complaints that could embarrass the target group, and cause them to solidify their opposition. Your group may earn a reputation for reasonableness, if you can achieve a resolution without the need for formal complaints.

"Accept that democracy works. It's messy, but it works."

AN ADVOCATE

23. Lobby decision-makers

Before you use this tactic, check with knowledgeable advisors about how far you can legally take it. Although individuals acting on their own behalf can pursue any type of advocacy, lobbying for specific legislation or political parties is off-limits to many non-profit organizations. The following actions, however, are not considered lobbying, and may be undertaken legally as part of any advocacy effort (Douglas & Claypoole, 1992; Swords, 1991):

- Communicating with or educating decision-makers and the general public about the general importance of policies (this becomes lobbying if legislators or the public are approached to vote a particular way on a specific bill or referendum);
- Advocating for specific policies being considered by non-legislative groups (e.g., retailer associations, school boards, state boards of health, public transportation authorities);
- Advocating for issues to such officials or groups as state attorneys general, regulatory authorities, administrative agencies, or police authorities;
- Advocacy aimed at government executives (e.g., mayors, governors) as long as you are not asking them to promote, discourage, or veto legislation;
- Public interest litigation or related judicial activities;
- Developing policy positions that are different from a specific legislative proposal;

- Testifying before a legislative committee (if the committee has requested testimony) or testifying on a subject that involves an organization's own self-defense.

Potential benefits

So-called lobbyists have great influence on the policy decisions made every day in this country—"if you can't beat'em, join 'em." Getting involved in lobbying and related activities can complement other advocacy tactics at your disposal.

Direct action tactics: Mobilizing public support

24. Sponsor a community conference or public hearing
25. Conduct a letter-writing campaign
26. Conduct a petition drive
27. Conduct a ballot drive
28. Register voters, or distribute registration material
29. Organize public demonstrations

24. Sponsor a community conference or public hearing

Open discussions about the issue and your advocacy campaign itself will increase community awareness. You will need an accessible public meeting place, and appropriate publicity, either through flyers, or the mass media, or other means. A respected speaker knowledgeable about the issue can be a good draw. Opponents might seize on an opportunity to disrupt such a meeting—but if that happens, it could result in negative publicity for their side, and positive attention for yours.

Potential benefits

You can gain visibility for your group, provide public education about its goals, and get an opportunity to recruit new members. This can also be a good way to get media attention.

25. Conduct a letter-writing campaign

This tactic involves encouraging large numbers of people to write letters to newspapers and/or public officials expressing support for, or opposition to, some development. Consistency is important, so your advocacy group should give the letter-writers a very clear statement about the type of message you want conveyed. It's also important to pay attention to the logistics necessary for carrying out this tactic—identifying targets to be contacted, specifying how they should be reached, and arranging for volunteers to recruit letter-writers. A word of warning: don't make any public announcement claiming success with your letter-writing campaign until it is over, because getting people to agree to write a letter is the easy part: getting them to actually do it may prove harder.

Potential benefits

This tactic can bring increased visibility for your issue. It's also an easy way to involve group members, and may bring in supporters from outside your main group.

26. Conduct a petition drive

A successful petition action, incorporating a clear objective, can demonstrate widespread community support for the changes you seek, and heighten public awareness of the issue. Such a drive is time-consuming, however. Once the statement is drafted and approved by the group, volunteers copy, circulate and return the petitions. Completed petitions are then distributed to appropriate decision-makers, and brought to the attention of the media.

Potential benefits

A petition can demonstrate broad support for the issue, and bring visibility to the group.

27. Conduct a ballot measure drive

Ballot measures allow citizens to participate directly in the legislative process through voting. These measures may take the form of referenda that in essence allow voters to veto legislation before it takes effect; or initiatives that offer voters the opportunity to pass new laws. State laws vary, but in general referenda qualify for the ballot by petition and are almost always seen at local government level. Initiatives are placed on the ballot by citizen petition *or* by elected officials. They may be referred to as binding advisory measures, meaning that the law must be enacted if approved by the voters. Petition-supported initiatives tend to occur at the state level, while binding advisory measures occur at the local level. Non-binding advisory measures are placed on the ballot by local elected officials (e.g., city council members or county supervisors). These measures allow the elected officials to get voter feedback on proposed legislation, but do not require any action.

Potential benefits

These tactics are not often utilized by health advocacy groups, but can be powerful ways to set and influence the public agenda. If successful, they typically have longer staying-power than other tactics.

> "90 percent of the politicians give the other 10 percent a bad reputation."
> HENRY KISSINGER

28. Register voters or distribute registration material

Provided that registration is non-partisan, advocacy groups can register voters without violating rules about political activity. They can also distribute voter education material, as long as it provides a non-biased presentation of the positions of all candidates, or all issues on the ballot. Political strategists have long used these tactics to give them a critical edge in local, state, and federal elections, using voter education and registration to increase voter turnout, as well as the level of knowledge about the issues.

Potential benefits

In addition to getting out the vote of those favorable to your position, taking an active part in politics can have another benefit: public officials will take you and your issue much more seriously when they perceive you as having influence over voters.

29. Organize public demonstrations

For this tactic, you call upon members and supporters to demonstrate their opposition to a target group through marches, parades, rallies, informational picketing, street theater depicting the target in various modes of villainy, and whatever else the imagination conjures up. Some demonstrations may be organized to ensure the target's normal routine will not be disrupted; others may have the intention of disrupting normal functions. Besides building pressure on the target, demonstrations can draw media attention to the group and the issue, raising the public's awareness.

This tactic requires careful consideration, especially if you intend to disrupt. When strong feelings are involved on one or both sides, demonstrations can become volatile and difficult to control, which can lead to violence or arrests. Before you organize a public demonstration, make sure it is legal: depending on local regulations, you may require parade or other permits. Ask yourselves these questions: What image is likely to develop for the group as a result of a public demonstration? What effect will it have on future dealings with the target? Will resorting to demonstrations split the membership? (See Chapter 8, "Dealing with the Opposition," for more on the subject of non-violence.)

Potential benefits

In addition to gaining broad public exposure for your issue, and generating public support (if all goes well), you should add to you group's sense of solidarity, commitment and empowerment.

Direct action tactics: Using the system

30. File a formal complaint
31. Seek enforcement of existing laws or policies
32. Seek enactment of new laws, policies or regulations
33. Seek a negotiator
34. Seek a mediator
35. Seek a fact-finder
36. Initiate legal action

30. File a formal complaint

With this step, the group makes an important commitment to the campaign. You are taking a public, official stand with respect to a grievance. The filing may be with an appropriate administrative body, or with someone who has authority to rectify actions done in the name of an organization. This action, especially when it follows unsuccessful "informal" efforts, underscores your resolve and likely will increase your visibility. You may be tested at this juncture about your intentions— i.e., you may be asked to spell out what you really want in order to settle the issue.

Filing a formal complaint frequently requires one or more persons to act as complainants. Documented evidence of the problem and its consequences will be necessary, at least within a reasonable time after filing the complaint. It is, of course, vital to have your facts straight, in the interest of the issue and your credibility. It is helpful to have knowledgeable advocates prepare the complaint, gathering the evidence and providing advice about procedures. If your group does not have its own resources, legal aid groups may be of help.

There can be downsides to this tactic. Once the issue is referred to responsible agencies, you may surrender some control over the terms of any settlement, and also over the time frame, as the complaint wends its way through the official process. There's another factor about which you can make no prediction: the target may respond with such strong denial and outrage that a very long battle results, leading, predictably, to the courts.

Potential benefits
You should achieve a fair hearing of grievances. Also, you will be on public record, underscoring the seriousness of the issue.

31. Seek enforcement of existing laws or policies

After you identify those responsible at the highest level for enforcing a law or rule, you seek negotiations for improved implementation procedures to ensure that the law or rule is adequately enforced. To carry out this tactic, you will need the following: a copy of the written law or rule; evidence that the law or rule is not being enforced, or is being enforced in a discriminatory fashion; and the identity of those responsible for enforcement.

Once you are armed with the facts, seek a meeting with key administrators to discuss appropriate enforcement issues. Further tactics clearly will be needed if the complaint is rejected, or if the response is inadequate, or if the enforcement process fails to correct the problem.

Potential benefits
Key officials are likely to respond to such complaints with at least a temporary crackdown, which might improve the situation for a while and provide the group with a sense of achievement.

32. Seek enactment of new laws, policies or regulations

Pursuing the legislative route, or otherwise calling upon decision-makers to address problems, can provide some solutions. In initiating this tactic, you may draft the proposed legislation or policies yourself, or encourage a respected decision-maker to do so, in addition to endorsing and pushing it. You will need to demonstrate that a problem, in fact, exists; that other efforts have been attempted, but have failed to correct the problem; and that there is wide support for the proposed solution. In addition to recruiting support within the legislative body, you will need to find constituents who will write and speak out in support of the initiative. If the proposal is controversial, you can expect some lively opposition.

Potential benefits
The legislative process may prove to be the best route for improving or eliminating certain problems. This tactic is likely to involve large numbers of people, and bring favorable publicity for the group.

33. Seek a negotiator

If you and your opponents become so alienated that you can no longer deal with each other productively, it may be worth while to find an experienced, successful negotiator. This person can arrange a meeting with the opponent on your behalf, and negotiate a settlement. If your group is genuinely eager to resolve differences, and avoid further risks and costs, this can be a good solution.

Potential benefits
As well as providing for conflict resolution, this tactic will demonstrate your group's reasonable efforts to resolve the conflict—contrasted perhaps with the other side's unreasonable posture.

34. Seek a mediator

Mediators differ from negotiators in that they are selected by both sides to assist them in reaching an agreement. Parties at an impasse over their differences may find a way out with help from a respected neutral third party skilled in negotiation. Mediators have no authority other than that given to them by the parties who request their assistance. Unless the parties agree to it, they may not even have authority to recommend solutions. Even with limited authority, however, an experienced mediator can be extremely useful, finding the hang-ups on both sides, and perhaps guiding disputing parties to a settlement that they were unable to see without help. Local judges, attorneys, or others involved in the legal system may be able to recommend mediators who meet your needs.

Potential benefits

If your group is the one to propose mediation, you will demonstrate your reasonableness and willingness to seek resolution. Mediation may also provide the best means for finding a useful resolution of your problem.

35. Seek a fact-finder

The fact-finder offers an additional means to help parties negotiate their way to a settlement. The fact-finder may recommend a solution to both sides. Neither side is obligated to accept the solution, but the process frequently provides for public release of the fact-finder's recommendation. The resulting public pressure might make it hard for either side to reject it. This obviously presents a risk, because you don't know in advance whether you will be able to live with the fact-finder's recommendation. If you can't, your advocacy group might incur considerable resentment, and make the public unhappy with your position and objective.

Potential benefits

If the result is one you can live with, you will demonstrate your reasonableness, and you will have found a solution.

36. Initiate legal action

Legal action is usually a last resort, not to be considered unless the target seems totally entrenched and unmovable by reasonable means. Court action requires one or more individuals injured by the defendant organization to be named as complainants, or plaintiffs. The objective is to rectify a condition, seek compensation for damages, and/or establish a precedent that will thwart similar action in the future. You will need an attorney from the beginning to provide counsel about the case, and oversee the gathering of evidence. Some attorneys will take civil actions on contingency—i.e., they agree to a percentage of damages awarded if the court rules in your favor. Otherwise, the process is likely to be costly in both financial terms, and in terms of the amount of work and time involved. Accurate predictions about the time-table of the process are difficult to make, because of legal maneuvers beyond the group's control—including the possibility that a verdict may be appealed.

Potential benefits
The threat of legal action alone may lead to settlement talks. If successful, litigation can prove valuable, setting precedents to clear the way for others.

Direct action tactics: Getting serious

37. Arrange a media exposé
38. Flood the system
39. Organize a boycott
40. Organize passive resistance

37. Arrange a media exposé

This involves giving one or more media representatives information potentially embarrassing to the target organization or one of its key representatives. The tactic is frequently one of last resort, because of its punitive nature—and because it is uncertain whether embarrassment will soften the target for favorable change. The tactic can also rebound. If there is anything inaccurate in your allegations about misconduct and improprieties, or other embarrassing revelations, you may end up in court. In addition, you may invite similar scrutiny from the opposition or from the media itself. Make sure that your group and its leaders can survive an energetic hunt for scandal. An additional pitfall is that the issue itself might get lost in the exposé. Also, your group may acquire a reputation for being radical and vicious.

Potential benefits
This is a quick way to gain the interest of the local media, and public awareness of the issue.

38. Flood the system

This is a concerted effort to demonstrate the failings of an unworkable system by overwhelming it, while remaining within the law. For example, targeting a restaurant, you might organize dozens of people to ask for non-smoking tables at about the same time. If a mass of people are waiting to be seated while empty tables are being held for smokers, management may be persuaded to make more non-smoking tables available. Or organize dozens of supporters to bombard local police with information on stores that sell tobacco to minors. As the evidence of illegal activity (and public concern) mounts, police may feel obligated to take direct action.

"Flooding the system" requires considerable planning, and the cooperation of a large number of people. Without those elements, the tactic may backfire and make the group look impotent.

Potential benefits:
This tactic can get results, and is also satisfying to group members.

39. Organize a Boycott

Boycotts require a large number of consumers to stop using a service, business or commodity until the provider meets certain conditions. The purpose is to get the provider's attention by way of his or her financial base. To succeed, you will need a just (and justifiable) cause, and a provider who can be financially or politically damaged by a well-organized boycott. Continued access to the media can be helpful in spreading the boycott.

It is advisable to get legal counsel if you have any doubts about whether a boycott is legal, or if there is any possibility that an organization or business might have legal recourse for damages resulting from boycott action. Even if everything is legally above board, a boycott is not something to be undertaken lightly. It is, after all, a declaration of economic warfare. Before embarking on this tactic, ask yourselves if such an action might alienate any economic interests that have supported you directly or indirectly. Does your group have more sympathy in the community than the target? Remember, too, that a well-organized boycott requires a good deal of time and energy, and might divert the group from other important tasks.

Potential benefits
A successful boycott can be very educational. Similar businesses will learn that negotiation with you is preferable to risking a boycott themselves. A boycott will also increase broad public awareness of your group and its issue, particularly if the action has been covered in the media.

40. Organize passive resistance

Drawn from the lessons of Mahatma Gandhi, Martin Luther King, Jr. and others, this tactic has members refusing to comply with laws, regulations or policies they consider unjust. The tactic is particularly beneficial when the community is generally sympathetic about the injustices, and is comparatively prosperous—in other words, they don't see your action as bringing any direct economic threat. One or

> "I don't know the key to success, but the key to failure is to try to please everyone."
> BILL COSBY

more committed, respected organizers willing to lead by example can be very helpful, and give others the courage to follow.

Passive resistance can sometimes proceed for long periods before it has any impact, and in some cases may never have much impact at all. Among other potential drawbacks are the loss of leaders, if they are arrested and jailed; the possibility that the group's official status might be jeopardized, or its resources used up in legal skirmishing; and the chance of negative reactions from the public, the decision-makers, and the media. After all, there's no guarantee that your action will be seen in a favorable light by others.

Potential benefits
This may establish the group's moral authority, and demonstrate your seriousness about the issue.

Selecting tactics

As we said at the beginning of this chapter, you should consider including as many tactics as are appropriate to your purpose, your position in the community, and your chosen strategy. Here are some final suggestions:

- Beware of becoming trapped in any one tactic. It can cause you to lose perspective, or can drain you of energy and resources.
- Beware of being sidetracked by mini-campaigns. For example, if a certain agency is slow to release data you need, it's tempting to launch a secondary campaign aimed at the offending agency—but that can deflect energy needed elsewhere. In such a case, your group would be wise to find the quickest means to gain access to the information it requires, and avoid getting hung up on damaged pride.

Tactics in the real world

To demonstrate how certain campaigns have put strategy and tactics together in the past, we have collected a number of case histories, which you will find in Chapter 11. From these accounts, you may develop your sense about which tactics are most appropriate to the circumstances. Are there any used in the case histories that you would have rejected? Are there any not used that you would have employed?

From those case histories, you can see how a campaign is put together as a gradual building project—how the advocates gear up, start to apply pressure, then react according to the response of the target, or according to the momentum of the developing campaign.

The bottom line: winning

Throughout its campaign, the group should be prepared to negotiate a settlement. Sometimes the timing may not seem right—for example, you might have just completed a successful fund-raising effort, or started to build up momentum in a way that the group finds exhilarating. However, the bottom line is that the issue that got you started needs to be resolved. So remember these two points:

1. You're not in this to do tactics. Your purpose is your objective. When and how it is achieved is often beyond your control.

2. At any time in your campaign, whether organizing, fund-raising, or even undertaking research, you should be alert for opportunities to bargain with the opposition, as a first step towards bringing the campaign to a conclusion. This is much easier if you don't get too hung up on the excitement of tactics. Stand back from time to time to re-examine your objective. Then you will have it in mind when—and if—opportunity knocks.

One final reminder: your campaign is dynamic and changing. You can't plan it out in every last detail at the beginning, but may often need to adapt your tactics (or develop new ones) to cope with whatever the opposition throws at you. That's covered in the next chapter, "Dealing with the Opposition."

8

Dealing with the Opposition

"It is wise in war not to underrate your opponent. It is equally important to understand his methods, and how his mind works. Such understanding is the necessary foundation of a successful effort to foresee and forestall his moves."

LIDDELL HART,
THOUGHTS ON WAR, 1944

Almost without fail, if you are on the right track, someone will object to your mission or your strategy. Opponents may press for an alternative, fight to keep the status quo, or even try to destroy your group. Hence, you become targets of *counter advocacy*, which may take the form of gentle persuasion, education, benign neglect, misunderstanding or even outright harassment. This chapter will help you deal with the road-blocks that your opponents attempt to place in your path.

In some cases, resistance may come from community leaders and decision-makers. Calls for reform can be sensitive subjects for them, because such demands can suggest that problems occurred on their watch. In other cases, people will resent what you are doing because they are, in fact, targets—and their resentment means that you are having an impact.

In any case, don't cringe at criticism. It's a key feature of this playing field. Listen to it, respond to relevant points, and strive to keep it from interfering with your objective. If you have proceeded responsibly, taking enough time to analyze the issue and clarify your objective, you will be sufficiently comfortable in your commitment to withstand criticism.

The opposition has an arsenal of responses, and there are many ways for us to respond to them. For the sake of your campaign, you have to know these counter-advocacy tactics when you see them, and know how to defend against them. It's part of effective advocacy. In this chapter, we present a framework for identifying the types of responses that opposition groups might make. We will also provide suggestions for responding.

Defensive strategies used by the opposition

Although the opposition's response cannot be predicted with certainty, there are some typical patterns have been identified. Lee Staples, in his book *Roots to Power* (1984), categorizes them as "The Seven D's of Defense." We expand that to "Ten D's and an S": *deflect, delay, deny, discount, deceive, divide, dulcify, discredit, destroy, deal* and *surrender.* A target may respond in any or all of these ten ways, perhaps shifting its response midstream, throwing advocates off balance. With advance preparation, advocates can be ready, shifting gears quickly to deal with whatever strategy the opposition chooses. We start with a description of those different opposition strategies. There you will find an analysis of why the opposition uses these strategies, and some guidelines for the techniques you can use to deflect or defuse them. (Some of the examples are taken from the field of environmental advocacy, but are broadly applicable in the field of health.)

1. Deflect

A common and natural response to criticism or attack is to sidestep it, and try to shift the focus of attention. This could mean diverting attention to side issues, or "passing the buck" to some group that has no effective control of the problem. The tactic is designed to turn your energies elsewhere.

Here is an example: your advocacy group demands clean-up of a hazardous waste site. Your opponent's response is to deflect your attention through an in-depth discussion of a general environmental bill caught up in congressional subcommittees. Or they might deflect the debate into one about jobs. Sometimes issues raised by the opposition are valid—for example, it may be true that an environmentally destructive program provides employment. But that does not relieve a corporation of the obligation to follow safe waste-disposal practices, and should not change your priorities.

Typically, "passing the buck" involves shunting the issue to a part of the target organization that has little or no decision-making power, such as the "community relations" department—or even to another organization. The target's objective is to frustrate your attempts to identify the responsible party. Knowing the decision-making process and who holds the power (see Chapter 3) can help you skirt this minefield successfully.

2. Delay

One of the most common responses for a target faced with substantial criticism is to engage in delay techniques. In this case, the opposition wants you to think the issue is being addressed, when in fact nothing is happening. By postponing dialogue or confrontation, the target seeks to diffuse the advocates' momentum, wear the advocates down, and ultimately remove the issue from the public eye. Successful delay can demoralize a group, producing a level of frustration that in extreme cases can cause members to vent anger at each other.

One all too familiar delay strategy is the formation of a "study commission" that has no real power to affect change. Bureaucrats may brush aside abundant data that's available to them, claiming it is insufficient. They may give the appearance of being generous by inviting the group to nominate some of its own members to serve on the commission—but in such cases, valuable time and energy are frequently wasted on committees and busywork. The billboard industry, for example, is notorious for setting up "sign commissions." Padded with industry lobbyists and representatives, these commissions remove the debate from the public eye and delay it to death.

3. Deny

An opponent may deny there is any validity to claims about a problem, or about proposed solutions. It may carry denial to the point of refusing to meet with the group, or by being "unavailable" for dialogue. Implicit here: there is no problem—or if there is a problem, it's too small to worry about.

Clever targets may disguise denial by saying they would *like* to help but, sadly, there isn't enough money in this or the next budget to do so. (There are traces of delay there, as well, implying you may want to come back in two years and try again.) Or they may try a "good-cop-bad-cop" approach: "I see your point, but my hands are tied. I'm only one small voice in this big organization."

One of the most flagrant examples of a denial strategy is the tobacco industry's claims that the evidence linking tobacco and health is controversial. The industry likes to say that there is a "statistical association" between smoking and disease but still denies that there is a causal relationship.

4. Discount

There are two main ways an opponent may discount you: by minimizing the importance of the problem, or by questioning your legitimacy as an agent of change. The target may seem to make token efforts at communicating with the group, while most of its energy is directed to downplaying the crisis. For example, in the case of the Three Mile Island nuclear power-plant disaster, officials minimized the gravity of the radiation leaks and the consequences (as some are doing to this day).

The tobacco industry uses discounting tactics when they question the relationship between smoking and disease.

Another method of discounting is to apply derogatory labels to advocacy groups, dismissing them as alien to the community, insignificant or "extremist" (i.e. radical, fascist, leftist, reactionary, etc.). Or the target may discount a group's claims by challenging its facts and figures (which underlines the importance of basing your campaign on a firm foundation of meticulous research). See also "Discredit" on page 90.

5. Deceive

Deception is conscious manipulation that may take the form of subtle tricks or lies. There are similarities between deceiving and denying, but deceiving is more conscious and intentional. For example, a target may deliberately attempt to mislead advocates into believing meaningful action has been taken or is forthcoming, when that is not the case. There may be feigned sympathy, but no sincere intent to engage in dialogue, to compromise, or even to consider the advocates' position. A deceptive tactic may be strikingly simple—for example, when an opponent with a "hardline" reputation offers angry advocates refreshments as a surprise gesture of good will, thus knocking them off balance.

Here are some examples of deceptive moves:
- A target organization offers to meet with advocates, but makes itself available only at times or places that are inconvenient enough to make such a session extremely unlikely, if not impossible.
- Meetings publicized as negotiations prove to be one-way information sessions. The target organization monopolizes the agenda with long explanations, complete with detailed charts explaining why it cannot meet the advocates' demands. "Dialogue" becomes lecture, and the advocates are rendered passive.
- Targets seek to confuse and intimidate advocates with a flood of jargon and bureaucratic red tape. The advocates begin to drown in legal, organizational, or technical explanations for why change cannot happen.
- Targets may present substitute "solutions" which do nothing to address the problem, but confuse and distract the advocates.
- Target organizations may draw upon bogus or manipulated surveys to derail advocates. For example, the billboard industry has been known to present a discredited public opinion poll to support its position for less restriction on tobacco and alcohol billboard advertising.

6. Divide

By planting dissension, the opposition wants to undercut advocates' unity, sowing enough discord to divide and conquer. One way to divide an advocacy group is to pit more militant against moderate advocates. For example, the opposition may make appeals for "level-headedness," encouraging moderates in the group to criticize more militant members. The opposition may also attempt to win over the more moderate leaders of a group by offering token concessions of small consequence, hoping to induce moderates to declare a victory and drop a cause before *real* concessions are forthcoming.

Targets also have been known to try "buying off" leaders of advocacy groups with offers of personal or professional rewards, such as salaried positions, or hefty financial offers for personal property.

Divide-and-conquer techniques are not directed only at advocate leaders. Targets strive at times to sow dissension between advocacy communities. For example, one technique in the hazardous waste industry is to pit one neighborhood against another. In that scenario, many groups end up battling each other to keep waste sites out of their own back yards.

Another technique is to establish a "front group" to compete for a constituency. While such groups appear to share the goals of an advocacy organization, they actually belong to the opposition.

The opposition may also try dividing residents of communities from advocates by organizing neighborhood "advisory committees." Ostensibly, these committees are set up to monitor complaints about offensive conduct by the target organization, and to give the target "advice" concerning the objectionable action. However, there is no mechanism for questioning the conduct of the target. (When such committees are established prior to the arrival of a hazardous waste site, you can assume that such a facility is indeed going to be built!)

By providing limited resources to alleviate a problem, target organizations can divide advocacy groups into those who want to get at least something out of the dispute, and those who want to hold out for more. A. H. Robins Co., manufacturer of the Dalkon Shield intrauterine contraceptive device (IUD), used this approach. The company provided cash compensation ranging from $125 to $725 to plaintiffs seeking legal redress for severe injuries, including infection, sterility and death, in the 1970s and 1980s. Literally hundreds of thousands of women were thought to have been injured by the product; the settlement offer severely split ranks between those prepared to settle, and those demanding more compensation.

"You have to be very self-motivated to enjoy your work—enjoy engaging in battles."
AN ADVOCATE.

7. Dulcify

A synonym of *dulcify* is *mollify*, which is to "soothe; pacify; appease." One way to do this is for an organization to dispense jobs, services or other benefits in response to a group's action. Thus, the situation appears agreeable in the short-term. Harsh criticism is warded off, and attention is diverted from long-term negative effects. For instance, a logging company marketing an environmentally unsound plan to a rural community emphasizes job opportunities. The short-term benefit of jobs may appear more concrete than long-term problems, such as diminishing forests and wildlife, an economy built on a rapidly depleting resource, and low wages for those new jobs.

A target organization can also give the appearance of agreement, while conceding little, by falsely assuring advocates that agreement is imminent. There may be attempts, also, to give advocates false expectations by agreeing to the mildest demands.

The line between compromise (which is often desirable) and dulcifying is sometimes vague. Advocates will need to be alert to the opponent's true intent if they are to chart an appropriate course.

8. Discredit

The opposition may spend much of its energy trying to undermine the group's credibility through the media, public hearings or direct persuasion. Discrediting is meant to cast doubt on an advocacy group's motives and methods. For example, the opposition may seek to label advocates as unreasonable, emotional, irresponsible, radical or communist. Advocacy groups may be described as consisting of a few "agitators" who are not representative of the community. The goal is to prejudice the public against a group, and to frighten the advocates themselves into "rational" (i.e., less threatening) action.

In some cases, the effort to discredit a group can be quite demeaning to its members—as when the opposition suggests that the advocates are out of step with society, and need to adjust their own values and attitudes. For example, members of a public housing tenant group may be encouraged to join "control your child" campaigns in response to their demands for adequate building maintenance. The implication is that the tenants, not the landlords, are the problem.

In other cases, the opposition may pack hearings with supporters to heckle and disrupt the proceedings. The point is to unnerve those calling for change, and discourage their potential supporters.

9. Destroy

A target may respond to an action with attempts to eliminate a group, or destabilize it so that it self-destructs. Through legal or economic means, or crude scare tactics, the target may directly attack the advocates' constituents, members, or organizational base. Stakes may be high, with much to be gained and, from the perspective of the target, much to be lost with respect to its vested interests. In some cases, advocates may inadvertently play into the hands of target organizations, giving them an opening through which to deliver the *coup de grace*. For example, advocates making unfounded or malicious accusations risk being sued for slander or libel, with devastating damage suits.

It is not unusual to see target organizations threatening lawsuits—not because they view the courts as a viable response, but to deter advocates from valid criticism. Their aim is to intimidate, causing the advocates to back off. In fact, the risk of being sued is not high. Although an exceptionally well-heeled target organization facing legal sanctions may counter-sue to force an advocacy group onto the defensive, such lawsuits are rare. In the grassroots toxics movement, the Citizen's Clearinghouse for Hazardous Waste found the odds of being sued to be about one in two hundred.

However, the *threat* of legal action can be a powerful weapon, and the opposition can gain an advantage without even having to proceed all the way to court. For example, "discovery" procedures preparatory to formal proceedings would entitle the opposition to relevant information about the advocacy group's operations. The advocacy group may be justifiably nervous about opening up important records such as telephone logs, and membership and contributors' lists. In addition, group members may be subject to "depositions" in which they are questioned under oath by counsel for an opponent. So the threat of a lawsuit alone may be a powerful deterrent.

The opposition may also try such tactics as economic sanctions, threats to fire group members, evictions, curtailment of credit or funding sources, or assaults on financial resources through legal battles. Some opponents may not be above obvious scare tactics, such as threatening physical violence or arrest. When a group is organized and knows its rights, however, such threats have little effect.

10. Deal

For a variety of reasons, a target organization may opt for the path of least resistance and offer to make a deal, working with the advocates toward a mutually acceptable solution. Dealing has obvious advantages: collaboration is likely to enhance mutual understanding. As defenses relax, chances for creative solutions improve.

However, some deals can deflect an advocacy group from its purpose without providing much of value in return. Compromising requires sharp attention to the economic, political, and social climate as well as to the dynamic among the players. (See "Know when to negotiate," page 97.) If you are not careful, compromise can be tantamount to victory for the opposition, leaving your advocacy group far short of its goal.

One example is the Comprehensive Smoking Prevention Education Act of 1984, a bill that required four rotating warnings to be printed on cigarette packs. From the point of view of the pro-health forces, this bill this was the result of a compromise: to secure its passage, they had to give up their demand for a reference to the addictive nature of smoking, and other more strongly worded warnings. However, compromise at one point in time does not mean that future improvements are out of the question. The issue of health warnings remains on the front burner of health advocates, and the warnings on cigarette packets are likely to be strengthened in the coming years.

11. Surrender

The best-case scenario is for the opposition to agree to an advocate group's demands. If this rare development occurs, it's important to remember, in the euphoria of the moment, that talk is cheap. A victory isn't complete until the opposition has followed through on its concessions or promises. In other words, the advocacy campaign is not over when terms are agreed to, but only when *all* the follow-through is complete.

Why the opposition responds as it does

Reviewing some theories from social psychology may be help you develop an understanding of why opponents respond as they do. It can also help you anticipate the actions or reactions of the opposition, and plot your own strategies.

In *Effective Social Action by Community Groups*, Alvin Zander examines the different perspectives that activists and target organizations may have with respect to change. The activists, who aim to reduce a source of dissatisfaction, have much to gain and little to lose. If they fail, it's rarely an embarrassment, because the objective was probably ambitious in the first place. Targets, on the other hand, have much to lose, regardless of their response. If they implement a proposal from advocates, they may not get any sense of accomplishment or pride, since the initiative was not their own.

Further, they may face the prospect of criticism from constituents or community members who believe the change to be unwise. Rejecting the proposal can also bring criticism, unless the idea is recognized as universally bad.

Zander lists three general ways targets are likely to respond to proposals for change:

1. Welcome the ideas of change agents

Targets most likely to respond to change are those not strong enough to withstand criticism. Targets are likely to welcome change:

- When it is seen as mutually beneficial;
- When both sides recognize as valid the other's point of view, and are eager to recognize similarities in goals;
- When the advocate group is non-threatening, and respects the autonomy of the decision-maker.

If those conditions are present, the target does not need to go on the defensive. The climate is fertile for compromise, or even surrender.

2. Oppose the ideas of change agents

A target may oppose the content of a proposal, claiming one of many possible reasons: it is illogical, unworkable, or immoral; it is based on invalid criticism; the solution would be too costly; the advocates do not represent community interests, etc. In this scenario, the target decision-makers want the activists to take "no" for an answer. At the same time, they want to avoid conflict, and might use delay and denial in the early stages to prevent conflict from developing. If the target does need to come right out and reject a proposal, it may try to explain its resistance in a way that invites minimum opposition from the activists. It may also try calming activists by offering token concessions with little substance, making the demands seem unreasonable—or the target may seek to postpone the decision indefinitely. (See "Deflect," "Delay," "Deny," "Deceive," "Dulcify.")

3. Resist the ideas of change agents

According to Zander, reasons for flat-out resistance vary widely: the target may feel advocates are seeking only their own benefit; the target may not accept the group's information; or the advocate group may have failed to clearly identify the problem. When targets throw up resistance, advocates respond with further resistance, giving rise to a circular situation. If the resistance-cycle is not broken by constructive problem-solving, and is allowed to build, the target may use more aggressive forms of resistance, including attempts to discredit or destroy advocate groups.

General guides for responding to the opposition

There are no pat formulas for responding to the other side, but you can start with this principle: you should always look for a strategy that fits the level of resistance from the opposition. It may be tempting to try a pre-emptive strike, hitting the opposition before it has mounted any major attack—but this is not usually advisable. While the element of surprise may be useful in some instances, forcing a target into the role of enemy before seeking a more civil or persuasive approach may blow an opportunity for negotiation, and could seriously damage your cause in the long run. Following is a partial list of techniques to guide your response, in line with the suggestions for "Advocacy 'Etiquette'" in Chapter 4.

A. Turning negatives into positives

"A strong offense in an organizing campaign requires being ready to counter any defense your adversary might employ," Lee Staples says in *Roots to Power*. Every attack presents an opportunity to turn what appears to be a negative situation into one where you gain the upper hand.

Responding to a lawsuit with a countersuit is an example of how tables may be turned. Discovery and deposition processes may give us the kind of information that can exert tremendous pressure on the target. If these processes produce public disclosures of potentially embarrassing information, this can strengthen a group's hand while, at the same time, forcing a target into a deeper defensive posture.

A small advocacy group that is being attacked in the courts by a powerful opponent can use the attack to attract sympathy, claiming that the legal assault is a draconian measure intended to bury the real issue. In some cases, the target can be shown as intent on depriving the group and others like it of their constitutional right to free speech, which is highly valued by most people in the United States. By framing an issue in terms favorable to your group or cause, even though in reality you might have suffered a setback, you may often get favorable press. For example, if you have lost a key city council vote on a health-related ordinance, rather than accepting defeat, you can talk about how this will provide fuel for further actions by health advocates. Or draw attention to the role that special interest groups (more powerful than good ol' citizens like you) played in defeating the ordinance. Or use the attention gained by the "loss" to promote your group or your group's cause to the community at-large.

Turning a negative into a positive is like counterpunching in boxing. A boxer does not simply block a punch. He responds offensively and instantaneously by attacking the opponent's unprotected or vulnerable area—like the ribs or the jaw. In advocacy, when targets attack they leave themselves vulnerable. We can respond proactively, instead of reactively, by spotting the vulnerable point and countering. There's another way of saying this: The key to dealing with trouble is for you to be the one who makes the trouble, rather than letting it happen you. And remember, what you learn in one defeat may be key to limiting future losses.

B. Going public with the opponent's tactics

There is a great deal of leverage to be gained by *labeling* the tactics used by the opposition. A tactic loses some of its power when uncovered for all to see. An example of this can be found in the way an advocacy group responds to the "divide and conquer" tactic. If advocates allow targets to play upon internal tensions, pitting them against each other, groups may turn their anger inward, and eventually self-destruct. Identifying the opposition's "divide and conquer" tactic as what it is may give renewed focus to the campaign. It can further strengthen the group by directing members' anger at the opponent, rather than at each other.

If a target responds to your demands by making token concessions, you can deflate this attempt by identifying the concessions for what they are—tokens. Not only does that maintain group focus on the objective, but it strengthens your hand in the campaign, assuring the public that a more favorable outcome is expected. (But make sure that the target's response is, in fact, a token. It could be very damaging to a campaign to stick the "token" label on a good-faith response, making the target justifiably suspicious about the group's motives.)

C. Framing the debate on *your* terms

If a target succeeds in getting you to discuss the matter on *its* terms, you have lost a significant measure of control. If you can avoid being forced on the defensive, you will gain an important edge. Thus, it is important to convey issues in terms that mesh with how *your* group thinks about it. If you cannot set the terms of the debate, it is advisable to at least not let the debate get out of control (i.e., don't get into a situation where you are constantly on the defensive, responding only to your opponent's arguments).

As we said in the last chapter, the ability to frame the debate on your terms is of vital importance to a number of tactical approaches. In the next chapter, we will give you additional suggestions for framing the issue as you reach out to the general public through the media. You need only look at how elected officials surround themselves with so-called "spin doctors" to understand the importance of framing—which can go far beyond choice of words. The setting can also "frame" an issue. For example, you could choose a forum for discussion that is uncomfort-

> "Even an ant may harm an elephant."
> ZULU PROVERB

able to the opposition, such as a "seminar" they sponsored on company grounds, or a debate in front of an unfriendly crowd, with television cameras present. For your part, you want to arrange for your meetings to be as comfortable for you as possible, ejecting any hecklers or disruptive members of the opposition—or making them feel uncomfortable. And if you invite guests from the opposition for a discussion or debate, have your best speakers there to counter them. Nailing down terms of any confrontation will increase the likelihood that the issue does well in the amphitheater of debate.

D. Balance and illusion

Responding to the opponent's counterattacks with what they don't expect can give your campaign an edge. The principal—balance—is the same as that applied in sports. In tennis, the accomplished player keeps the opponent guessing with a variety of shots and placements—short, long, cross-court, top-spin, back-spin, lob. No single response can be anticipated. In many forms of athletic competition, the ability to "mix it up" is a definite plus. Similarly, keeping opponents off balance in health advocacy is crucial to disrupting their rhythm, momentum, and sense of timing. Because they cannot confidently anticipate and prepare for your moves, they are effectively deprived of an important edge.

Don't rely on set strategies. If you always stage a sit-in whenever decision-makers refuse to make concessions, for example, not only will the impact of this action diminish, but the target will grow increasingly efficient at blunting its effectiveness. It's better to respond with a wide repertoire of techniques making it tougher for opponents to predict your actions.

In this vein, nonviolent direct action, in and of itself, is an effective tactic for keeping the target off balance, and limiting repression. This is because while most systems and jurisdictions in this country are familiar with responses for squelching violence, they are knocked off stride by nonviolent actions. (For more on the use of nonviolence, see "G: Political jujitsu" on page 99.)

Illusion, similar to balance, goes one step further. The idea is to trick the opponent into wrongly guessing your intentions. In the world of magic, smoke and mirrors and similar techniques are used to draw the observers' attention to the wrong place, setting them up for deception. Using parallels again with sports, you can see how an edge is established with the play-action fake in football, the disguised forehand in tennis, the dink shot in volleyball, the curve and change-up pitches in baseball, and the feinting techniques in martial arts. All constitute the use of illusion for overpowering opponents.

A nice example of this tactic in action occurred during a television "debate" between a tobacco industry representative and Richard Daynard, a law professor at Northeastern University, and head of the Tobacco Products Liability Project. Professor Daynard was recruited to speak out against smokers' rights. He knew that the task would not be easy. (As the physician/activist Alan Blum points out: "Debating the tobacco industry is like wrestling with a pig. You both get dirty and the pig loves it.")

As the debate began, and the tobacco industry representative took the familiar party line about protecting the rights of smokers, Daynard realized that arguing against smokers' rights might be ineffective for two reasons: first, everyone was expecting him to do it, so the opposition had adequate time to prepare counterarguments. Second, it meant accepting the way the media and the tobacco industry framed the issue, rather than the way that an activist might frame it. Daynard decided to come out in support of smokers' rights—but with a slight twist. The rights he favored were the rights of smokers to sue tobacco companies for their disease. The interviewer and tobacco industry representative were so taken aback, so unprepared for this line of reasoning, that Daynard had the debate won in a matter of moments. The lesson? Keep your opponent off balance. Frame the debate in your terms.

You can also call upon illusion to create an impression that you have many more resources than you do, or are planning more actions than is the case. This can force opponents to prepare for several different situations, thereby diluting their response to what you eventually do. Saul Alinsky, the Chicago-based community organizer who carried confrontational techniques to new heights, said: "Power is not only what you have, but what the enemy thinks you have."

E. Know when to negotiate

To negotiate, in the context of advocacy, is to strive to settle a dispute. The process almost always involves compromise—not to be equated with capitulation or surrender. As a party to the negotiations, you have a right to participate in establishing the ground rules.

Opportunities for serious negotiations with the opposition may be rare and fleeting. More than likely, they will be delicate. You will be well-served to watch carefully for favorable signs that a chance for negotiation might be in the offing, because these chances may not be repeated. With experience, monitoring the climate for negotiation becomes easier (it's extremely useful to have someone with experience on your side). For example, buried in a target's otherwise belligerent statement about your campaign might be a hint about possible discussions: a spokesman might be quoted as saying of your group, "Since they are so irresponsible, I doubt they would consider meeting with us." In the face of such posturing and the emotions it tends to arouse, the signal about a possible meeting can be missed, and the opportunity lost. But here is an opportunity that should be seized: the chance to sit down with the other side indicates your group has achieved respectability and standing. It is a welcome development when the target reaches out in any fashion.

As you saw from the chapter on tactics, advocates can benefit greatly by probing for negotiation opportunities. Many tactics are ways to test the wind for various possibilities that might lead to negotiation, such as a chance to participate in planning sessions; the development of formal communication mechanisms; and so on. Of course, you can undermine the chance for negotiations. One way to do that, paradoxically, is by proposing talks prematurely. Such overtures may be viewed as weakness on your part, possibly closing the door to negotiations for several months.

Within the delicate art of negotiation, compromise is the most fragile element. In *The Consumer Movement*, R. N. Mayer provides a sense of this dynamic: "In any negotiation, one can err either by compromising too readily, by giving up ground that one could have easily won with a little more persistence, or by being too unyielding, with the result that the negotiations break down and an opportunity for mutually beneficial exchange is lost."

Effective advocates will be constantly aware of the dynamic between themselves and the other party, as well as the political, economic and social context of the talks. If, for example, the social tide is increasingly supportive of anti-tobacco efforts, the health lobby will have a stronger hand to play in battling the tobacco industry. Alternatively, where the public feels heavily dependent on tobacco for economic security, the health lobby might accept compromise in the interest of its constituents.

F. Consider your opponent's psychology

In *Effective Social Action by Community Groups*, Alvin Zander sees actions along a spectrum from "permissive" to "pressuring" or "constraining." Examples of permissive actions include presenting a plan for addressing a problem, or working with the other side in problem-solving. Constraining approaches are those that are combative and coercive (e.g., a boycott, physical harm, etc.). "Like behavior tends to beget like behavior," Zander maintains. Hence, targets tend to respond to advice, argument, intervention or aggression with advice, argument, intervention or aggression. This tendency is modified by how much the target likes or dislikes the proposed change.

If a target is seeking solutions to a problem, advocates may have an opportunity to join the target in the effort, and, in that instance, permissive methods can reduce resistance. Activists can further avert or diminish anxiety for the target organization by defining problems without immediately suggesting solutions. This shows respect for the target's autonomy. If and when the advocate group does propose solutions, advocates can soften these by proposing a tentative "trial period" so decision-makers do not feel fenced in.

Of course, such civil and permissive methods won't always work. You may have to resort to pressure tactics. Like mules averse to gentle persuasion, and immune to logic, some target organizations are more likely to accept change when hit on the head with a two-by-four, in the form of sit-ins, boycotts or other disruptive tactics.

When it does prove necessary, the pressure option is a longer road than the persuasive one, for many reasons. Targets are less likely to focus on the proposals than on the pressures being brought to bear, and their natural reaction is likely to be anger and resentment. If there is change, it will be in overt behavior: underlying beliefs will probably not be affected. Intensifying pressure increases the likelihood of heightened resistance, which will require more intense pressure, and so on. The feasibility of rational dialogue will diminish and the dispute may require help from a neutral process, like mediation (Zander, 1990).

G. Political jujitsu: Turning opponents' assets into liabilities, nonviolently

Gene Sharp gives us the term "political jujitsu" in *The Politics of Nonviolent Action* to describe how the opposition undermines its own power. This phenomenon finds the opponent's greatest asset, its superior power, being transformed into a liability. "By combining nonviolent discipline with solidarity and persistence in struggle, the nonviolent actionists cause the violence of the opponent's repression to be exposed in the worst possible light," Sharp says. "This, in turn, may lead to shifts in opinion and then to shifts in power relationships favorable to the nonviolent group." Examples where political jujitsu has operated successfully include the campaign in India for independence from the British Empire, the American Civil Rights movement, and the defiance campaign in South Africa.

Social change groups tend to have much less power and authority than opponents such as corporations, government agencies or legislative bodies. Activists have less access to the commercial media, fewer financial and expert resources, and less access to decision-makers, and they do not have the police to enforce their decisions. That's where "political jujitsu" comes in. It allows the activists to use the power and superior force brought against them to their own advantage by bringing disfavor upon the system, or tripping it up.

How? Activists persist with nonviolent discipline until the system responds heavy-handedly, out of exasperation or frustration. The common result is a shift in public sympathy, with other social groups and forces surfacing to work with the activists. You will find this is especially true when the opponent's policies are hard to justify.

Persistence is a necessary element of political jujitsu, because the process may require substantial time. At the outset of nonviolent direct action campaigns, it is not uncommon for the community to react negatively to the activists. By their very tactics they are different, and thus candidates for suspicion. They may be labeled as "agitators," and blamed for any violence that does occur. In these early stages, supporters of change frequently split between the nonviolent militants and the more conventional reformers or moderates. Thus, there is often initial polarization, which may even bring the opponent some *increased* support. For the activists, this polarization period is one of the most critical parts of the process and it is crucial to the efficacy of their strategy that they avoid actions that might confirm negative prejudices about them. It is primarily during this time that those negative prejudices will be magnified or invalidated.

As the activists persist with their nonviolent discipline, maintaining solidarity, the violence of the system is exposed and rendered increasingly repulsive to the general public. Shifts begin in favor of the nonviolent group. Eventually, assuming the activists hold to their discipline, the scales are tipped, and the shifts in power relationships accelerate, leading to widespread opposition to the system and support for the resisters.

Political jujitsu causes shifts by operating among three broad groups:

1. Uncommitted third parties
The sight of people enduring severe repression because of a belief in a principle is a moving one that is likely to affect previously uninvolved people. This can be true on local, national, or international levels. For example, British repression of nonviolent Indian demonstrators swayed world opinion toward the Indians.

2. The opponents' usual supporters
When opponents employ violence against nonviolent demonstrators, there is a higher likelihood that they will arouse opposition in their own camp. Violent repression is hard to justify in the face of nonviolence, and thus is likely to be seen as unreasonable. Also, it is easier for members of the opponent group to express misgivings when activists remain nonviolent. When members of the opponent group start to question the means of repression, they may also begin to question the cause. Dissent within the opposition's own camp can range from discomfort to criticism of opposition tactics, all the way to positive efforts to aid the activists. This was true in 1963 when nonviolent resistance by Buddhists in South Vietnam drew harsh repression from the pro-Catholic govern-

ment regime. Reacting to this brutality, massive segments of the Catholic population withdrew support from the government.

3. The general grievance group

The ability to withstand repression can be related to a strong conviction in the rightness of a cause, the courage to withstand intimidation, and the capacity to bear suffering. While repression often reduces the number of nonviolent activists, it can strengthen the will of those resisting. Numbers, in nonviolent action, are not as important as strength and persistence.

With time, of course, opponents grow more adept at responding to nonviolent action. They may use less violent means of repression to blunt the effects of political jujitsu. This does not mean the cause is lost. The grab bag of nonviolent tactics is huge, and includes economic sanctions in addition to political, social, and psychological pressure. And if opponents reduce the violent repression, or refrain from it, new doors open for other kinds of conflict resolution. (See Sharp: *The Politics of Nonviolent Action.*)

H. Concentrate strength against weakness: Insights from military science

Military science provides basic lessons about concentrating strength against an opponent's weakness for substantial gain. Although health activists may not feel comfortable borrowing from this source, military theory includes some tools that can be applied in health advocacy by either side. Hence, it's helpful to consider them, not only for your options, but in thinking defensively about your own "exposed flank." As you review the following concepts, think in terms of advocacy campaigns as much as possible.

Concepts of military strategy

Because the principle of war involves concentrating strength against weakness, a useful strategy is to create the appearance that your forces are being dispersed, which in turn causes dispersal of enemy forces. When that happens, concentration of force will be more likely to succeed. A fundamental error is giving opponents the freedom and time to concentrate to meet *your* concentration.

One military theorist says perfect military strategy produces a resolution without serious fighting (Liddell Hart, 1944). Hence, the point is not to seek battle, but a strategic situation so obviously advantageous that if it does not produce a decision, the battle surely will. The process develops defeat in the mind of the opponent even before battle is joined.

Here are three more attributes of a good strategy:

- **A good strategy involves economy of force.**
  A very small group avoids squandering its resources against a large troop when, instead, it can husband them for a balanced battle at a time more to its advantage.

- **A good strategy seeks to diminish resistance both physically and psychologically.**
  You can diminish resistance physically by exploiting time, topography or transport capacity to restrict enemy movement. This might mean a change of front, or a separation of forces, or measures that endanger the enemy's supplies; or you can menace the enemy's routes of retreat. Measures that restrict freedom of movement will also have a psychological effect. The opponent is demoralized when feeling trapped, or at a disadvantage.

- **Good strategy exploits the line of least resistance and expectation.**
  Apply physical and psychological dislocation before "throwing your weight" into a move. You want the opposition sufficiently disorganized or demoralized as to be unable to evade your action, when it comes. By thinking like your opponent, you can successfully visualize where resistance will be lower.

In terms of health advocacy, a good strategy for disorganizing the target, and lowering its resistance, is distraction. Drawing their attention to other matters clouds the issue for the opponents, and limits their freedom of action. For example, you can keep the opposition off guard and thoroughly distracted by maintaining multiple objectives, and a variable plan that is designed to confuse. Numerous minor coups and threats cause more distraction than a few major hits. Remember, however, that tactics of distraction are a means to an end. At some point, forces must be concentrated to achieve the objective.

Guerrilla tactics and counter-insurgency

Because the opposing sides in conventional war frequently share relative parity, analogies with advocacy are somewhat limited. Advocacy groups tend to be much smaller than their opponents. A more fitting comparison for the advocacy group, in this context, is with a guerrilla force, while the opposition might respond with its counter-part—counter-insurgency.

History demonstrates that successful guerrilla insurgencies had some things in common: great respect for superior force; refusal to meet that force on a battleground of the opponent's choosing; the ability to erode the will of the opposition physically and psychologically; accomplished techniques for demoralizing and distracting the opposition; the use of indirect rather than frontal approaches; and concentration of strength against weakness at crucial times.

For its part, the opposition might respond with the classic tactics of counter-insurgency, traditionally used by powerful bodies such as governments to head off guerrilla warfare. In *Counterinsurgency: Some Problems and Implications*, Edgar S. Furniss, Jr. delineates the difference between positive and negative counterinsurgency. On the positive side would be improvements in conditions that cause the need for guerrilla action to evaporate, while a negative example might include repressing the rebel groups with such tactics as espionage, sabotage and selective terror.

Similarly, a large organization can rely on positive or negative action to ward off attack by an advocate group seeking change. Positive action includes coopting the advocates' cause, and making concessions designed to win loyalty. Negative action would include tactics designed to discredit and destroy the advocacy group. It is useful for advocates to be able to ascertain whether conciliatory offers are being made in good faith, or as part of a long-term strategy to destroy the group.

Finally, here are two last military analogies, concerning learning from one's mistakes, and making sure of victory:

- Obviously, it is good strategy to learn from mistakes. An attack should not be renewed along the same lines once it has failed. Two similar setbacks will be very costly, not only in terms of resources but also because of the lost confidence experienced by the losing side.
- Military theorists recommend that victories be exploited. When opponents are defeated in war, victors want them to stay that way. There is a parallel for health advocacy. When a target organization is brought to terms, you should leave no doubt about the results, exploiting the victory to the fullest. The object is to keep buried a problem that required so much time and commitment to bury.

Summary

In advocacy, every response leads to a counter-response: the group that can guess the nature of the opposition's counter-response will be ahead of the game. Even though the process may be hard and time-consuming, it will be well worth your while to put yourselves in your opponents' place and anticipate their moves. You will then avoid being taken by surprise, and can make your next move in this advocacy chess game with calm deliberation.

9

Using the Media

This chapter will describe the use of media and public relation tactics in support of health advocacy. Effective use of the media can be important to your success in a number of ways:

- The media can increase decision-makers' and the public's knowledge of the issue, and put it on the public agenda;
- The media can help change attitudes, and mobilize support by framing the issue on your terms (see Chapter 7, page 61);
- The support of the media can provide a valuable weapon in your armory, by bolstering your standing in relationship to the opposition;
- When used in conjunction with other advocacy tactics, the media can also influence community health norms.

As you will see, most of our suggestions are for media coverage through news programs, talk shows, features, and editorials. At the end of the chapter, we will include some tips for incorporating public service advertising (PSAs), "small" media, and word of mouth in your campaign.

Preparing a media campaign

As politicians and businesses know very well, media campaigns cannot be left to chance. Careful preparation is key. It is important to think through your media campaign—in the context of your overall strategy—well before you issue your first press release, or invite the media to your first demonstration. This will mean:

- Researching the local media to find out which newspapers, TV channels or radio stations reach the audience you most want to affect, and which people in those media outlets will be your best contacts;
- Preparing consistent themes and messages that frame your message in a positive light, and give continuity to your campaign;

- Incorporating media plans into your overall strategic plan, so that major campaign events can be designed (when appropriate) with media requirements in mind;
- Carrying out your campaign with the sort of confidence and professionalism that shows the media you mean business.

Researching the local media

Even before you have specific plans for stories, assign volunteers to research local media outlets. They should listen to the radio stations, watch the TV programs, and read the newspapers. It is helpful to compile information about the outlets in a "media inventory" that can tell you at a glance whom to approach to fulfill different needs—especially at the outlets that reach the largest numbers of people, or the people you most want to affect. Here are the main questions to which you will need answers:

- **What is the audience for each of the media outlets?**
  Your researchers can call the media outlets directly to find out their audience composition and their reach—the geographical area covered.

- **Which news reporters are assigned to cover the type of story that you might generate? Which editors or producers might be most sympathetic?**
  On a large newspaper or TV station, many reporters specialize, either because they are assigned to a certain beat, or as a matter of personal interest. The media outlet can tell you who these are. As the campaign progresses, personal contact will become particularly important. Some of your best media coverage might come about because an advocate can pick up the phone and tip off a friendly reporter or producer about a breaking story.

- **Which feature columns or talk programs might offer in-depth coverage of the issue?**
  In addition to the news stories, you should consider the possibility of getting much longer and more in-depth coverage—for example, through features in different sections of the newspaper; on television interview shows or news magazine shows; or on call-in or interview programs on radio. You will greatly increase your chances of getting extensive exposure if you can demonstrate to producers and editors that you are familiar with their output, and are able to tailor a presentation to suit their audience and their interests.

- **What are the important deadlines for the programs or newspaper editions that you most want to appear in?**
  Knowledge of the nuts and bolts of the business will help you choose the most convenient time for press conferences and staged events.

■ **Which newspaper or broadcast editorial boards might be most receptive to the idea of officially backing your issue, and run editorials in your support?** Knowing what type of issues have won editorial backing in the past can give you guidance about whether to make a formal pitch to an editorial board to win endorsement. (If the outlet is owned by a conglomerate with links to the opposition, or is dependent on advertising over which the opposition may exert some control, your chances may not be great!)

Choosing the channel of communication

A comprehensive media campaign attempts to use as many channels of communication as necessary to get broad coverage, and to demonstrate clout. However, media outlets all have their own advantages and disadvantages, and may need to be approached or used in different ways:

Television is an excellent way to reach a lot of people at once. Formats include news stories and series; public affairs programs; talk shows; editorials; and paid advertising. Stations also run free public service announcements (PSAs), but these may be expensive to produce, may not be aired while people are awake, and may not be shown at all if they seem controversial.

Many communities now have opportunities for using public access television, and these are worth exploring. However, public access programs are not widely seen, and thus require a major promotion program to attract an audience.

Radio has a number of formats similar to television, but is often more accessible, and may provide a better way to reach your audience. This is especially true if you want to reach subgroups of the population, such as teenagers or members of ethnic groups, who may form the predominant audience of certain stations.

In some communities, call-in talk shows on radio carry a good deal of influence, and can be helpful in setting the agenda. If you need to advertise a specific event or program, radio may give you a reasonable placement for free PSAs.

Newspapers can offer spot news coverage, such as a single story on a particular health topic, or multipart news coverage, such as a series on teenagers and gang membership. Editorials, letters to the editor, op-ed guest columns, and even editorial cartoons are also good ways to get your message across, if the paper chooses to give you this type of support. Other sections of the paper such as those devoted to sports, business, or lifestyle may offer opportunities for more detailed information in feature stories.

Neighborhood newspapers are an excellent way to reach a targeted audience, and especially valuable if you are addressing neighborhood concerns such as placement of tobacco billboards.

Keeping up the contact

Personal contact is of vital importance in media relations. The gatekeepers at all levels are more likely to do you a favor if they know who you are. Early in the campaign, designate one or two people as your media contacts. These may or may not be the people who conducted the initial research (see above) or who serve as your spokespeople (see below). They should be knowledgeable about the media, because it is they who will set up press conferences, put their names on press releases, and help reporters find stories or photo opportunities.

Here are some suggestions to help those contact people establish a good working relationship with the press.

- Stay in touch! For example:
  - Instead of mailing press releases, drop them off in person (pick a time when the editor or reporter is not close to a deadline, and may have time to talk);
  - If there's a national story breaking, phone the reporter who covers that beat and ask if he or she would like your organization to provide an exclusive local angle;
  - Hand out Rolodex cards with the name of your organization's main expert. This makes it easier for reporters to call for information whenever your issue is in the news.
- Make a point of thanking the media people who help, or who produce stories about your organization or issue. Write to their superiors to praise their contribution.
- Don't complain if your material is not used—though it's OK to ask how you can improve your chances next time.

Choosing your spokespeople

Before launching a full-scale media campaign, your group should select one or two spokespeople. By limiting the number of spokespeople to one or two, you will help the press, and the public, to put a name and a face to your issue, and will ensure that your message is consistent. Also, your spokespeople will become increasingly adept as they get practice in speaking to the press, or appearing on interview shows.

Choose your spokespeople with care:

"We must figure out how we can make an impact on society without being one of the power players. The more you can get the public involved in the issue, the greater the likelihood that you will succeed."

AN ADVOCATE

- They should be deeply committed to your issue, and should be prepared to learn about it in depth, so that all the facts and arguments that might come up in an interview will be at their fingertips;
- They should enjoy talking in public, and be good at it;
- They should be available, often on short notice, in case a major story breaks;
- If possible, they should be known and respected in the community—a well-known physician, for example, might be an excellent choice.

Preparing your message

Before you go public, you should frame your message in a format that the media can use most efficiently, and that will be most effective. Your goal is to enable the general public to understand your issue, and to put your "spin" on the facts of the case, counteracting the arguments that your opponents may use (see Chapter 7, page 61, for examples of "framing the issue" in your terms.)

Experts recommend that you select three to five main points, and plan to stress them consistently. You should make those points the centerpiece of interviews or presentations, and return to them in any debate with opponents. Most news coverage will allow you space or time to make only these few points. It is in your interest to make sure they are well-developed and punchy. Here are some suggestions for distilling complicated data into "media bites" that will help convey the information you want:

- If you need to use complex statistics, use "social math" to bring the numbers to life. For example, rather than giving a death rate of 1,000 or so in numbers, say it's the equivalent of two jumbo jets colliding and crashing with no survivors.
- Use striking images. For example, point out that making part of a room smoke free is like chlorinating only one end of a swimming pool.
- Localize an issue with statistics that apply to your community: be prepared with brief local case histories to illustrate your point. "One woman in Green Acres waited fifty-three minutes for the police to respond!"

You have your issue. You have your spokespeople. You have your main points and your counterarguments all ready. You know which press outlets you most want to carry your story. How do you put it all together? In the following sections, we give suggestions for getting news coverage, making use of editorial opportunities, and preparing for interviews.

Gaining access

Broadly speaking, there are four ways you can get news coverage of your issue:
- By staging a newsworthy event
- By holding a press conference
- By issuing press releases
- By feeding stories to individual reporters, feature writers or producers.

The newsworthy event

As you saw in the chapter on tactics, a successful advocacy organization often has the potential to generate events that news media enjoy covering. The media are always on the lookout for good, strong stories, especially if there is a photo-opportunity involved. They pay attention when groups of citizens use imaginative tactics (for example, "Flooding the system," No. 38). Many direct action tactics can be planned with the media in mind, or you can build in elements that are likely to attract the attention of both the media and the public. One excellent example was the action taken by a group of teenagers in Solano County, California, who purchased over 250 packages of cigarettes or smokeless tobacco in an undercover buying operation. The media were then invited to watch the teenagers throw the tobacco into a hazardous waste container, which was then prepared for disposal at a hazardous waste site. The media coverage was excellent.

When you plan an event that you hope will make news, send out notices to the press ahead of time to tell them what will be happening, when and where. Have your spokespeople ready to answer their questions, whether or not you combine the event with a formal press conference.

The press conference

Press conferences should be used very sparingly. They are a nuisance for the media to attend, and if nothing very newsworthy emerges from your first, you may find no one comes to your second. In general, press conferences should be held only if you have significant, dramatic, timely and/or controversial news to announce; if you produce people who are too interesting or important for the press to ignore; or if you have a tremendous story in human interest terms.

If you decide to hold a press conference, here are some rules of thumb:
- Hold the press conference in the morning, to get the best coverage.
- Notify editors and broadcast news producers several days in advance. Remind them with phone calls the day before the event.

- Prepare press kits containing background information and a press release (see below).
- Have the press sign in. If any important people are missing, call them later; hand-deliver press kits, and offer to arrange interviews.
- Pay attention to logistics. Choose a quiet location; provide maps so everyone can find you.
- Pay attention to setting and drama. You'll get most coverage if you can produce more than "talking heads." For example, have teenagers in project T-shirts talking about their experiences, or people giving emotional accounts of disasters or achievements.
- Limit prepared statements by your spokespeople to one or two, of no more than five minutes each, then take questions.

Press releases

Press releases, like press conferences, can wear out their welcome if they don't give the media something they can use. Keep them for when you have something new to announce—and think of ways to make the story more attractive by building it around additional "hooks." Can you announce a milestone, such as the first time a community event is sponsored by a fruit juice company, rather than a brand of beer? Is this an anniversary? For example, the anniversary of a particularly violent crime could provide a springboard for the announcement of a crime-prevention initiative. Can you use a seasonal event or holiday as a peg? High school graduation can provide a framework for stories on drunk driving, or New Year's day for a press release on health-related resolutions. Is someone of prominence involved? Can you provide a local human interest angle? Giving a human face to a story gets the message across better than a recitation of facts (though be careful not to let your story be drowned by one individual's perspective).

Once you have a solid story for your release, give it a professional look by following these guidelines:

- Use stationery that shows clearly where the release is coming from (a banner heading with the name of your organization in large type is better than regular letterhead).
- Use a headline that explains what the release is about. Don't try to be cute—that's the newspaper's job.
- Double space the text; leave generous margins; use only one side of the paper, and don't use more than two pages.
- Write the story as an inverted pyramid, with the most important information first. If only the top half or third or even fifth of what you've written is used, it will still make sense.

- Make the opening paragraph no longer than three or four lines, and include information about "who, what, where and when."
- Either write, "For immediate release" or, "For release on (date)."
- Include the name and telephone number of one or two people who can be contacted for additional information.

Dealing with individual reporters

Being a resource for good story ideas is one of the most important things you can offer media organizations. Don't assume that they are brimming over with stories concerning your community. Quite often, they are actively looking for new local ideas, and in some communities rely increasingly on dependable help from knowledgeable people.

Your best media coverage may come from in-depth reports or features set up through your relationships with the individual reporters or producers. As your campaign progresses, your designated media experts should develop contacts with members of the press, and suggest stories to them. (In some cases, your campaign may develop such momentum that the reporters and TV producers call you for ideas!)

Using the editorial sections

Editorial sections can help your campaign in two ways: giving you free exposure, and/or giving you the endorsement of the newspaper or the broadcast station.

Editorials

Newspapers and some broadcast outlets will give their editorial endorsement to certain local events or campaigns. To encourage this, ask if your spokespeople can make a brief presentation at one of the regular meetings of the editorial board. Even if a paper does not print an editorial supporting you, it may provide space for your views on its op-ed page. Many TV and radio stations provide opportunities for people to deliver their own free speech messages.

Letters to the editor

Letters to the editor can help spread your message—but use them sparingly, making one strong point at a time.

Letters can be used to demonstrate the strength of your group, especially if you orchestrate a letter writing campaign around some burning issue. They won't all be printed, but the editor will get the message. Sometimes, thank-you letters to the editor will also be appropriate.

Interviews

Interviews come in two types: those you initiate, and those that are set up by the media outlet. In either case, whether the interview is for broadcast or for a newspaper, make sure your spokesperson is prepared. He or she should have:

- Background knowledge about your organization and campaign;
- Knowledge of the issue, including any controversy about it either locally, regionally or nationally;
- The three to five basic points that you want to stress;
- Knowledge of what counterarguments may be made during the interview, and how to refute them.

Your spokesperson should also watch the program that he or she is going to appear on, or read articles by the reporter doing a newspaper interview. This person should also practice, with a member of your group taking the part of the interviewer, and asking the hardest questions that might come up.

Brief the reporter or interviewer

If there is time, always give the interviewer background information, and ask about the direction the interview is likely to take. Although they don't like to give you their questions in advance, interviewers will usually tell you about the ground they expect to cover, and, in the case of a broadcast, who else will be on the program.

Watch out for traps

The press loves controversy, and may try to get you into a defensive position, or invite you to attack an opponent. Stay calm. Try to avoid the appearance of being angry, embarrassed or surprised. If someone makes an outrageous allegation, correct the facts, but don't attack the people who distorted them.

It is wise to have another member of your organization present at all interviews. If the interview is later distorted during editing, this person can help you get the record put straight.

Experienced advocates suggest that you don't tell a reporter anything "off the record." Most will respect your wishes, but the risks are too great if they do not.

Other channels of communication

Ultimately, your choice of media should be dictated by the audience you want to reach. To get your message across, you may need to go beyond the confines of the news. Whom do you want to reach, and how can you reach them? It may be that educational videos have a role in your campaign, reaching people in community clinic waiting rooms or at community forums. Employee newsletters could be a good vehicle, or small ethnic papers. In some cases, you may want to consider advertising.

Advertising

If you are given free space (for example, on buses or billboards) or free air-time (on TV or radio) you may have little control over the way your message is disseminated. It's all too common for TV PSA's to go out in the middle of the night. If it is extremely important for you to make an announcement that will reach a high proportion of the population (for example, if you are announcing an upcoming event) then it might be worth your while to buy newspaper space, or air-time (radio is usually a better bargain than TV for this purpose.) Also, strategically placed paid ads in buses, rail transit cars or waiting areas could support your efforts.

Print products

In addition to using the mass media, you may want to incorporate smaller printed pieces into your campaign, such as brochures describing your mission; booklets or handouts to help individuals make behavior changes; flyers or posters anouncing events.

Even though there are probably people in your group who are handy with their computers, and feel they can make adequate materials themselves, it is wise to consult a professional graphic designer. People pay more attention to materials that look good.

One problem with print products is their distribution. Leaving them in doctors' offices or other public settings is usually not sufficient. You may have to get out to places such as movie theaters, laundromats, beauty or barber shops, grocery stores, retail outlets, libraries, places of worship, music stores, malls, worksites, schools—wherever the people you want to reach congregate. In some cases you can solve the distribution problem by adding your message to something that is already widely distributed, such as telephone book advertisements, yearbooks, souvenir programs, restaurant placemats, grocery bags and carts, or paycheck envelope inserts.

One possible resource for distribution is the human being, who can act as a walking (or driving) billboard. T-shirts, visors and caps are good places for messages. Bumper stickers can also provide excellent exposure.

Word of mouth

For many communities, word of mouth may be the most effective communication channel, especially for the so-called hard to reach people who do not receive information from TV, radio, newspaper or print messages. These groups may put the most trust in information from those they socialize with on a regular basis. Social clubs, sports leagues, boys and girls organizations, school clubs or educational organizations, religious and political groups, neighborhood associations, fraternal organizations, boards and committees, local merchants and business associations are all good channels. The point is to be creative about where you advocate your message.

Summary

To sum up: put your message in as many places and in as many formats as possible, based on knowledge of where your audience gets its information, and how you can best harness the power of local media. The idea is not only to influence policymakers and community decision-makers, but also to change the general population's perception about health-related issues. Do not, however, compartmentalize media activities, or segregate them from the rest of your campaign. No matter how many column inches or broadcast minutes you achieve, your media campaign is unlikely to be effective unless media use is integrated into broader project plans.

Sections of this chapter are partially adapted from *Media Advocacy For Tobacco Control* by Linda Weiner, published by the Stanford Health Promotion Resource Center with funds from the California Department of Health Services, Tobacco Control Section (1994).

10

Evaluating Health Advocacy Organizations

"If at the end of an advocacy event the people cannot replicate it for another cause, if there is a continued reliance on outside experts, then the project has failed."

AN ADVOCATE

How are we doing? What have we accomplished? Evaluation provides health action groups with information that can assist internally and externally. Internally, you can learn ways to improve the management of the organization, while you can also document successes for external funding sources, and for others essential to the group's survival.

Evaluation can be done at a number of different levels. At one extreme are the complex measures of success that require analysis by specialists. At the other extreme is the group that sits around at the end of a campaign and discusses what happened, asking each other if they did well, or if adjustments should be made to correct the course of their efforts. In this chapter, we are assuming that your needs will lie somewhere in between. At the end of the chapter, we include worksheets and simple record sheets that can be used by people without specialized training. These may not fit with all your particular needs—but at least they may provide a starting point for evaluation of your efforts.

As you will see, in some cases evaluation plans begin with decisions about what you want to measure, and these decisions must be made at the start of the project. In Chapter 5 ("Making Your Plans") we reminded you that objectives should be measurable—so you can prove what progress has been made. If your selection process followed the guidelines we gave, your job at this stage will be that much easier.

We will give examples of three types of evaluation, under the headings of Process measures; Outcome measures; and Impact measures.

Process measures

Process measures provide information about how a campaign is going. How smoothly is it running? Is it achieving expected levels of community support, financial support, publicity and so on? Five measures of process may be of particular value to advocacy organizations, their constituents or their funders:

1. Community participation

Under this heading, you might count the number of people participating in public forums, committee meetings, marches, rallies and other events sponsored by the group.

Keeping track

You can keep track of figures indicating participation and support by way of sign-in sheets, and accurate membership records. Prepare ruled sheets with columns for recording dates, names and addresses.

2. Media coverage

The amount of media coverage can be measured by the number of column-inches of space in newspapers, or minutes of television and radio time devoted to the issue, the organization or its activities.

Keeping track

Designated members of your group can complete logs monthly. See page 125.

3. Financial resources generated

Success can be measured not only in terms of grants, contracts or donations received, but also such resources as "pro bono" professional services, or facilities provided by other organizations.

Keeping track

Monthly logs should be completed by members of the group. See the "Funds and resources" record sheet on page 126.

4. Members' satisfaction ratings

Although you may gather a general idea of member satisfaction during the course of the project, it is wise to conduct more formal surveys at intervals to check on their satisfaction with leadership, planning, and other aspects of group process.

Keeping track

See "Members' satisfaction survey" on page 127.

5. Analysis of critical events

The impact of events is hard to measure quantitatively, but you can gather valuable qualitative data from those involved with your issue or campaign. They can give you useful perspectives on key events in the life of the advocacy organization.

Keeping track
Structured interviews should be conducted toward the end of the project, when they can also serve to provide information on outcome and impact. See "Format for key participant interview" on pages 128-129.

Outcome measures

Outcome measures give you information about specific changes or achievements that have occurred in the community as a result of your program. In addition to providing a record of major achievements, outcome evaluation can also help you detect small victories on the path towards fundamental change.

The following six outcome measures can help give your group information about specific achievements:

1. Services provided

How many new classes or workshops have been held in the community? Has the advocacy organization provided newsletters or other informational channels for its membership, or for the community? What new service programs are in place?

Keeping track
Logs can be completed monthly by group members (see the "Ongoing services log" on page 130).

2. Community actions

In this category, keep track of actions through which your group had an impact on those outside the advocacy group—for example, dealings with the mayor of your community, or street demonstrations, or undercover buying actions to show the availability of tobacco to minors.

Keeping track
These (and community changes in the next category) can be recorded on an "Event log" like the one on page 131.

3. Changes in Programs

It's important to keep track of community-wide changes in programs, policies and practices as they relate to the group's goals and objectives. Include those brought about by law enforcement, business, schools, city government, and other community sectors. To keep track of programs, record any new services established, such as workshops for young people, or home delivery of meals for seniors, or a homeless shelter. You might include formal changes in policy, such as new fines for drinking in public, or bans on certain types of billboards. Also write down any improved practices, such as increased vigilance to prevent drug dealing near schools. Even if the victories are individually small, they should be recognized as important outcomes for the organization.

Keeping track

Use the "Event log" on page 131 to record dates of changes. Keep it up to date with monthly entries.

4. Ratings of Significance of Outcomes

Here, members rate the significance of the changes you have carried out, in relation to the mission of your group. By looking at the changes that rate high, compared with those that rate lower, your organization can concentrate future efforts where they will have the most impact.

Keeping track

See the sample "Advocacy outcome survey" form on page 132.

5. Access to services

In this category, you record increases in the actual community services related to your group's efforts. For example, if your program involves the need for more drug treatment, or contraceptive services for adolescents, you should record increases in the number of clients served by specific agencies. Sometimes such figures are hard to obtain—in that case, additional advocacy efforts may be required to pry them lose from the responsible agencies.

Keeping track

Increases in services can be shown in graph form, like the sample opposite.

6. Objectives met over time

The number of objectives met may be hard to measure, but it is worth your while to try, because the data may provide solid evidence of achievement for both your group and others, such as your funding source. As you remember from Chapter 5,

Sample measure of access

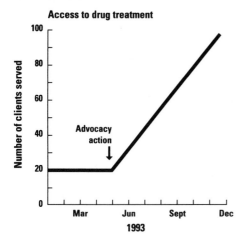

Sample measure of objectives met over time

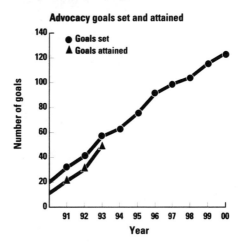

"Making Your Plans," one of the criteria for a good objective is that it is measurable. At this stage, this will prove very valuable, as you review the objectives you set up when making your action plans, and compute the percentage of community change objectives that have actually been achieved each year.

Keeping track
A graph can show what percentage of objectives is being achieved. See the sample above.

Impact measures

Impact measures provide information about the ultimate effectiveness of the advocacy organization. In other words, have you achieved actual change? Are people in your community breathing cleaner air, or getting less smoke in their lungs, or choosing not to drive drunk, or getting access to the care they need, or getting more nutritious school lunches, or postponing pregnancy in adolescence, or finding alternatives to gang violence?

Whether or not you can measure such changes depends, of course, on whether you had a firm baseline to start from—and that is one reason why a thorough base of knowledge about your issue is so valuable. Only when you know what the teenage pregnancy rate was before your program, and how the change relates to that in similar communities, can you consider claiming any success from an apparent reduction.

Any significant success you can measure at this level will bring rewards in the form of announcements you can make to the media, and hence the community. Such successes will also bring you respect in the eyes of other organizations and agencies in the community, and may be valuable in your efforts to secure additional funding.

Two types of measures may be useful in assessing the impact of advocacy efforts:

1. Behavioral measures

You can gather reports of changes in behavior, or sometimes observe them directly. For example, are community residents smoking less? Is there less sexual activity among teenagers? Are low-income senior citizens eating lunch more regularly? Data on individual behavior is not easy to gather, but may be obtained by administering surveys such as the *Youth Risk Behavior Survey*, or various modules of the *Behavioral Risk Factor Survey*, which are both obtainable from the Centers for Disease Control and Prevention in Atlanta (see Additional Resources, pages 161-162).

Keeping track
It is useful to display data in graph form, like the sample graph for showing behavior change related to preventing adolescent pregnancy (see opposite).

2. Community-level indicators

You can get information on certain changes in the community by studying the reports of appropriate community agencies. For example, if your issue involves alcohol abuse, one indication of change might be a reduction in the number of single vehicle accidents at night; another might be the number of complaints about rowdy behavior being made to the police. If your issue involves youth violence, the number of emergency room visits by teens or young men might provide a good indicator.

Keeping track
Finding sensitive and accurate data may require the cooperation of local and state agencies, such as the office of vital statistics in the state department of health. In other cases, local agencies such as the police, the school district, the Chamber of Commerce, or the local hospital can supply figures. Once you have statistics, you can demonstrate progress in graph form. (See sample opposite.)

Sample behavior measure

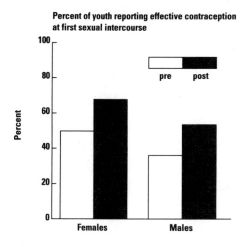

Percent of youth reporting effective contraception
at first sexual intercourse

**Sample community-level indicator for
substance abuse or injury control coalition**

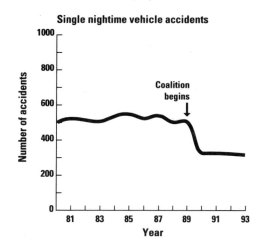

Using the evaluation

The main purpose of an evaluation is not to make judgments about the organization's efforts, but to find out how to make improvements in the organization itself, or the way it relates to the community. Collecting volumes of data that can only be understood by statisticians will not be helpful: an evaluation should, above all, be useful. If you hire professionals to help you with the evaluation, they should understand this fact. The final product should be something that both the leadership and the membership of the organization understand and use, while also meeting any requirements of funding agencies.

A good evaluation will help the group do the following:

■ **Celebrate accomplishments**
  Data regarding community changes may give the membership reason to celebrate small (or large) victories. Celebration can extend to announcements of achievements through the media.

■ **Make adjustments and contribute to renewal**
  If the data show that you have not achieved as much as you hoped, this may suggest specific adjustments in strategies and tactics. If you find that

levels of community action are not what you expected, this may suggest the need for renewed efforts to expand participation in your organization, and increase the energy level of those within it.

■ **Secure and maintain resources**
Evidence of community change and improvement will help you to add to your resources, by attracting new members, making new alliances with other organizations, or securing new funding.

In addition, the process of gathering information will help you educate key informants in the community about your purposes, and gain support for your issue.

This chapter is adapted from the following primary sources:

1) Fawcett, S. B. and Associates. *Evaluation Handbook for the Project Freedom Substance Abuse Prevention Replication Initiative.* Work Group on Health Promotion and Community Development, 4086 Dole Center, University of Kansas, Lawrence, KS 66045.

2) Fawcett, S. B. and Associates. *Evaluation Handbook for the School/Consumer Sexual Risk Reduction Replication Initiative.* Work Group on Health Promotion and Community Development, 4086 Dole Center, University of Kansas, Lawrence, KS 66045.

Media coverage

For use with Process Measure No. 2

Note: recorders should attach copies of articles

Name of recorder			Reporting period

Date	Topic of coverage	Paper or station	No. of inches/minutes

Funds and resources

For use with Process Measure No. 3

Dollars obtained, resources generated

Grants, contracts, in-kind donations

Date	Source	Amount

Members' satisfaction survey

For use with Process Measure No. 4

*Members should circle the number that best shows their satisfaction with each aspect
of the organization, and add their own comments if they wish.*

		VERY DISSATISFIED				VERY SATISFIED
Planning and Implementation						
1.	Planning process used to choose the organization's objectives	1	2	3	4	5
2.	Follow-through on organization activities	1	2	3	4	5
3.	Strength and competence of staff	1	2	3	4	5
Leadership						
4.	Clarity of vision for where the organization should be going	1	2	3	4	5
5.	Strength and competence of organization leadership	1	2	3	4	5
6.	Sensitivity to cultural issues	1	2	3	4	5
7.	Use of the media to promote awareness of the organization's goals, actions and accomplishments	1	2	3	4	5
Services						
9.	Training and technical assistance	1	2	3	4	5
10.	Fundraising and grant-writing	1	2	3	4	5
11.	Information and referral	1	2	3	4	5
12.	Advocacy	1	2	3	4	5
Community involvement in the organization						
13.	Participation of influential people from key sectors of the community	1	2	3	4	5
14.	Participation of people of color	1	2	3	4	5
15.	Diversity of organization membership	1	2	3	4	5
Progress and outcome						
16.	Progress in meeting the organization's objectives	1	2	3	4	5
17.	Success in generating resources for the organization	1	2	3	4	5
18.	Fairness with which funds and opportunities are distributed	1	2	3	4	5
19.	Organization's contributions to the goal of: _____	1	2	3	4	5
Overall approval rating:		NO				YES
21.	Is the community better off today because of our health advocacy organization?					

Format for key participant interview

For use with Process Measure # 5

Use plain paper for your notes, after gathering the following information for each participant interviewed

---

Organization

Participant

Participant's position

Participant's involvement with the organization

Date of interview

Interviewer

Part 1
Interview Process

INTRODUCTORY QUESTIONS TO IDENTIFY CRITICAL EVENTS:

- What key events or incidents were critical to the organization's development?
- What key events or incidents were critical to the organization's major accomplishments or successes?
- What key events or incidents were critical to the organization's setbacks or challenges?

When you have listed events in each of these three categories, circle events that seem particularly significant, and ask if the participant agrees with your choice. Analyze those events using the questions in Part 2.

Part 2
Analysis of critical events

For each of the critical events that you have identified in Part 1,
have the interviewee answer the following questions:

Name of event   **Date of event**

RATIONALE

- Why was this event particularly important?

CONTEXT OR CONDITIONS

- What was going on at the time of this event?
- What made the conditions right for this to happen?

KEY ACTIONS AND ACTORS

- What key actions brought about the critical event?
- Who were the key actors?

BARRIERS AND RESISTANCE

- Were the group's actions met with barriers or resistance?
- What types of barriers?
- Who resisted?

KEY RESOURCES

- What key resources (people, financial resources, political influence, etc.) were used to bring about the critical event?
- How were these resources used to overcome barriers and resistance?

CONSEQUENCES FOR THE ORGANIZATION

- What were the consequences (or results) of the critical event for the organization?

CONSEQUENCES FOR THE COMMUNITY

- What were the consequences for the community?

OVERALL LESSONS

- Overall, what lessons have you learned from your involvement with the organization?
- What lessons have you learned from the organization's attempts to define and act on its mission?

FUTURE DIRECTIONS

- What issues does the organization face in the future? What challenges should be addressed?

Ongoing services log

For use with Outcome Measure # 1

List all classes, workshops, newsletters, screenings or other services provided to community members.

Site _____ Recorder _____ Reporting period _____

Month/ year	Service	Location	Number served	New service? Yes / No

Event log

For use with Outcome Measures # 2 and 3

Use one copy of this form to keep track of each major event or action in your community relating to your issue. Include changes in programs, policies and practices.

Site	Recorder	Reporting period

TYPE OF EVENT, CHECK ALL THAT APPLY

☐ **New/changed strategic plan, committee, etc.**
☐ **New/changed program or service**
☐ **Action to bring about new program or service**
☐ **New/changed policy**
☐ **Action to bring about new policy**
☐ **New/changed practice**
☐ **Action to bring about new practice**

DESCRIBE EVENT BELOW

1. **Who did what?**
2. **What happened as a result?**
3. **Why was it important?**
4. **What organizations collaborated?**
5. **What community sector or objective does this relate to?**
6. **Was this the first time the event happened?**
7. **Other pertinent information**

Event:

Advocacy outcome survey

Sample Format

This sample uses a youth violence initiative as an example. Adapt it for your own purposes for use with Outcome Measure # 4

This survey lists four community changes. For each survey item, please circle the number that best describes how important the change is to the organization's mission of reducing youth violence using this scale

VERY UNIMPORTANT				VERY IMPORTANT
1	2	3	4	5

COMMUNITY CHANGES

Establish graffiti removal program

1	2	3	4	5

Change policy regarding punishment for drive-by shootings

1	2	3	4	5

Establish after-school program for 20 at-risk youth

1	2	3	4	5

Establish school-business monitoring project for 100 high school students

1	2	3	4	5

11

Case Histories

This chapter gives you a handful of case studies illustrating advocacy in practice. At the end of each case, you will find a list of some of the tactics used, and the numbers under which you can find those tactics more fully described in Chapter 7.

Case 1
The pay-as-you-go ambulances

The problem

Ambulance company drivers in Fort Smith, Arkansas, frequently demanded that sick patients pay immediately for the ambulance service, and some patients were harassed in the hospital until they paid.

The issue

To institute a pledge card payment plan for the ambulance company.

Background

Conway Ambulance Service Co. experienced financial difficulties, and was taken over by a young man and his wife who committed themselves to its success. However, continuing a practice from previous ownership, drivers routinely demanded that patients pay immediately for the service. The drivers had been instructed by their employer to tell families that the drivers would not be paid at all unless they received payment at the hospital. Drivers frequently intimidated patients, and refused to leave the hospital until payment was made.

The advocate group and its objective

ACORN was a local advocacy group that decided to address this problem. In reacting to difficulties facing clients of the ambulance company, it established two objectives:
1. To obtain a commitment from Conway to immediately bring sick patients to the hospital without consideration of payment;
2. To stop the harassment of patients.

Strategy and tactics

ACORN began by collecting accounts of Conway's conduct at neighborhood meetings. It researched the ambulance company to better understand its problems, and also conducted research to identify possible regulatory options. They found that in spite of the problems people had experienced, the community was generally sympathetic to the new owner of the ambulance company, because he was perceived as honest and concerned about providing decent service.

Given this, ACORN altered its initial strategy, which had been to attack the owner's integrity. The group did not want to alienate the community, local officials and the media. They devised an alternative strategy, which called for all sides to cooperate.

Actions

Having requested a meeting, seven members of ACORN visited the company owner, and both sides discussed their grievances. ACORN proposed that billing by mail was preferable for all concerned. The owner complained about low frequency of payments and rising costs. However, he was willing to explore anything that would increase the paid-up percentage while not alienating the community.

Following this meeting, the group devised the ACORN Ambulance Pledge Card System, under which the family pledged to pay its bill and the company pledged to stop demanding money at the hospital.

This system was presented to the owner at a meeting in the ACORN office, attended by thirty-five people from the community. The meeting had been scheduled by ACORN in the evening, to attract the largest number of people—including media representatives. The meeting began with several individuals recounting unpleasant personal experiences with ambulance drivers. Thereafter, an ACORN representative described the pledge card plan and proposed it as a solution. The owner declined to sign the plan then, but said he liked it, and would present it to the company board of directors.

On the next day, an article appeared in a local newspaper reporting that the owner supported ACORN's plan. The article placed the owner in a favorable light, and, as hoped by ACORN (which had briefed the newspaper in advance), made it difficult for the company to reject the plan. Besides the newspaper article, there was also television coverage of the meeting. While the owner was upset about the media coverage, he could not publicly complain, because ACORN only praised him.

Outcome

Private negotiations between ACORN and the ambulance company began after the meeting and continued for about one and a half months. The company agreed to the pledge plan on a trial basis, provided it was restricted to ACORN members. If the plan was successful, it would be extended to church groups, fraternal organizations and other community organizations.

Evaluation

A well-organized local group challenged a hostile payment collection system with an intelligent, aggressive campaign. Having established that the plan would benefit both sides, ACORN pursued the objective with imagination and good timing. Researching one's opponents paves the way for effective strategy. Here, while ACORN intended to lobby for the pledge card system by attacking the owner, it gave due weight to research showing the owner to be a diligent man who could gain sympathy from the media and local officials if attacked. It changed course.

Meetings organized by ACORN offered the owner very little control over the agenda. ACORN outnumbered the owner in the meetings, keeping him on the defensive. (This is a calculated risk. Outnumbering the opposition or otherwise taking them by surprise can be counterproductive. The other side may walk out, ending the meeting abruptly and jeopardizing further dialogue.) ACORN also used the media to its advantage, first by interesting them sufficiently to get coverage and secondly, by publicly heaping praise on the owner after the second meeting, which put him in a difficult situation.

Analysis of tactics

The following tactics were used (not necessarily in this order). See "Advocacy Tactics," Chapter 7, for more information.

Tactic 1   Conduct studies of the issue
Tactic 6   Document complaints
Tactic 9   Give personal compliments and public support
Tactic 14   Offer public education

Tactic 16   Postpone action
Tactic 17   Establish an alternative system or program
Tactic 19   Criticize unfavorable actions
Tactic 22   Make a complaint

Case 2
Medical services for the poor in California

The problem

Medical services were insufficient for indigent residents of Orange County, California, resulting in a high incidence of diseases that could have been cured or mitigated with proper medical care.

The issue

To improve medical services for indigent residents of Orange County.

Background

At the time this problem was addressed in Orange County in the 1980s, approximately one quarter of its two million residents were members of racial minorities, including hundreds of thousands of immigrants from Mexico. Altogether, about 200,000 residents lacked any medical insurance.

In 1975, the University of California, Irvine, bought the county's only public hospital, and the new UCI Medical Center (UCIMC) continued to serve more than 60 percent of the county's medically indigent. In 1981, however, reduced government funding for indigent care prompted the hospital to institute a policy of upfront cash deposits. Reforms in 1981-82 in the state's medical aid program for the poor further complicated care for the indigent. The state had tightened eligibility requirements, increased patient co-payments, and reduced physician reimbursements. Responsibility for the care of the medically indigent was transferred from the state to the county, and state funding was cut by 30 percent.

Orange County, which did not operate a comprehensive clinic for people over five years of age, was 56th among 58 California counties in per capita health expenditures from local funds. The Indigent Medical Services Program (IMS) only provided services deemed to "protect life, to prevent disability, and to prevent serious deterioration of health." Applicants faced a seven- to eight-week waiting period for medical care after submitting extensive personal financial documentation. IMS required large co-payments, and had low reimbursement rates, creating uncertainty as to whether services would be covered. These factors discouraged physician participation. Participation by the poor was further limited, because the program received little publicity.

The advocate group and its objective

UCI medical students organized a conference in 1985 to examine IMS and the responsibility of the county and the university for indigent medical care. Shortly thereafter, the Orange County Task Force on Indigent Health Care convened to pursue the issues raised in the conference. The task force included UCI faculty physicians, residents, and students; other health professionals; administrators of community clinics and hospitals; county employees; church people, and members of a variety of civic and social service organizations. It had a nucleus of twelve activists who met monthly and coordinated strategy, and about fifty others ready to respond to initiatives from the leadership. Members of the task force worked as concerned individuals rather than as representatives of organizations; they were not constrained by organizational considerations from adopting extreme advocacy positions or confrontational tactics, if needed.

The task force adopted the following objectives:
1. To document local obstacles to access, and the failures of current policies;
2. To lobby county government and local health care institutions to improve access;
3. To advocate on the legal front to put additional pressure on the financial barriers to medical care.

Strategy and tactics

Research was aimed at local access problems, with emphasis on studies that could rapidly raise the consciousness of county residents through the media and other sources, thereby improving the political climate for change. Initial strategy, aimed at decision-makers, highlighted IMS staff, the county board of supervisors, and the director of the Orange County Health Care Agency. On the legal front, attorneys in the task force and local law centers representing indigent clients encouraged the indigent to testify before the board of supervisors about violations of federal and state health program regulations.

Actions

The year 1986 was a very active one for the effort, on the following fronts:

- In the early months the task force began applying political pressure on the county about funding, eligibility and access to the IMS program. Initial efforts included private meetings with IMS staff, with aides of the board of supervisors, and with the director of the Orange County Health Care Agency. At these meetings, the task force documented the adverse impact of financial barriers on medical care. The sessions established a dialogue that later helped to improve access for the poor at local institutions.

- The task force began presentations at county budget hearings to raise awareness and inspire reform. Its early effort included a request for funding to support community clinics for people with no access to IMS, Medi-Cal, and other county health programs.

- Responding to cost-cutting measures by UCIMC that imposed financial barriers to care, the task force put a human face on the consequences by presenting testimony about specific patients unable to overcome these obstacles.

- The task force actively opposed efforts by UCIMC to attract for-profit corporations to buy or manage the hospital, because the corporations refused to assure continued access for uninsured patients.

- The task force coordinated the activity of a community coalition that fought repeated cost-cutting attempts by UCIMC to close or restrict access to its two satellite clinics, and its pediatric clinic.

- A series of studies documented access problems of the indigent, and the effect of these on their health.

- A population-based survey showed that the poor in the northern part of the county had very low utilization rates of preventive services, and were three times more likely than the national average to lack health insurance.

- Findings of the various studies were released frequently through news conferences and news releases, and were timed to coincide with journal publications or county budget hearings.

- Task force members joined with the Orange County Coalition of Free and Community Clinics in monthly meetings with the IMS staff to lobby for additional clinics as IMS providers.

Outcome

The combined research and media effort increased public awareness about the issue. There was a threefold increase in the number of approved applications at IMS, and an increase of 140 percent in the number of paid claims. This dramatic improvement followed two major developments:

1. The county replaced cumbersome eligibility documentation with declarative eligibility;
2. Additional clinics were included as contractual IMS providers.

Some administration and faculty members voiced opposition to the campaign on grounds that involvement by the university in indigent care would mean greater deficits, which would adversely affect teaching programs. However, UCIMC acknowledged the coalition by dropping recruitment of corporate involvement, and continuing to manage the hospital itself. Similarly, the campaign was credited with UCIMC's reversal on plans to make cutbacks, to impose financial barriers at two satellite clinics, and to close its pediatric clinic. In response to a task force press release, and testimony to the Board of Supervisors, the board investigated health care for the poor.

The Board of Supervisors and Orange County Health Care Agency increased county-funded prenatal care by one-third.

Evaluation

Countywide medical advocacy can induce significant improvements for the medically indigent. Here, indepth research was extremely beneficial. It demonstrated that a significant number of patients at UCIMC with access to primary care were unable to obtain further appropriate medical services because of financial barriers. Research was also used to identify alternative solutions.

This campaign was described in the *Journal of the American Medical Association*, where those evaluating it cited several concerns:

- As a strategy for addressing the problem, litigation is extremely costly and time-consuming.
- The advocacy strategy of the Orange County Task Force on Indigent Health Care was defensive, based on attempts to maintain services at a minimum level in the face of threats of cutbacks and barriers to access. Such a defensive posture will not contribute to more creative or proactive programs that would improve health care.
- While the task force lobbied against cutbacks at UCIMC, there was no evidence it appreciated the fact that the medical center was deeply in debt. The campaign to address the needs of the indigent ignored the economic root cause that led to greater stress for the poor. While there were short-term gains, these were unlikely to contribute to a cohesive health care system. (Authors in the *Journal of the American Medical Association* stated that a national health program was necessary to ensure universal entitlement.)

- The advocates' strategy did not involve making any apparent attempt to work with the medically indigent for change. Rather, the strategy consisted of publicizing issues and altering policy to increase access, based on the assumption that growing awareness of the availability of services would increase their use. Evaluators pointed out, however, that any strategy that can contribute to effective change—i.e., in national policy—must provide for empowerment of the indigent. When an indigent community is motivated by the prospect of going on the offensive to achieve reform, the underlying energy is overwhelming. Thus inspired, a movement can sustain itself because those likely to benefit are fervent for change.

Analysis of tactics

The following tactics were used (not necessarily in this order). See "Advocacy Tactics," Chapter 7, for more information.

Tactic 1	Conduct studies of the issue
Tactic 4	Request accountability
Tactic 12	Establish contact and request participation
Tactic 14	Offer public education
Tactic 19	Criticize unfavorable actions
Tactic 20	Express opposition publicly
Tactic 24	Sponsor a community conference or public hearing
Tactic 31	Seek enforcement of existing laws or policies

Case 3
The mentally ill of Maryland

The problem

Mentally ill citizens and their families received a disproportionately small share of state financing in Maryland, resulting in instances of neglect on the community level.

The issue

To advocate for greater priority with respect to state funding for mentally ill citizens and their families.

Background

Four Maryland citizens' organizations formed the Coalition for Citizens with Long-Term Mental Illnesses in 1983 to promote the development of a comprehensive, community-based mental health care and support system. In this, they were part of a national effort. By 1988, there were nearly 1,000 such grassroots groups and advocate organizations nationwide, made up of former patients of mental health services and their families, and affiliated with the National Alliance for the Mentally Ill (NAMI). In addition, the National Mental Health Association (NMHA), the nation's oldest mental health consumer advocacy organization, had 600 state and local affiliates. This organization, whose membership includes consumers, families, concerned citizens and professionals, is a leader in advocating for progressive community services, nondiscriminatory insurance, housing policies and other protections.

The advocate groups and their objective

There were four Maryland groups engaged in this venture:
1. The Alliance for the Mentally Ill of Maryland, a group of eighteen support groups composed of mentally ill persons and their families and friends;
2. On Our Own, an association of former residents of psychiatric facilities;
3. The Maryland Association of Psychosocial Services, an organization of forty nonprofit providers of community rehabilitation services, plus those who use these services and desire to be independent;
4. The Mental Health Association of Maryland, an educational, advocacy and service agency made up of citizen volunteers.

Common concerns about needs of the mentally ill and their families drew these groups together. The coalition narrowed its focus to citizens with long-term chronic mental illnesses, and established a goal of getting more state funds for community services. The initial priority was a $3 million increase for community-based housing and psychosocial rehabilitation programs.

Strategy

Because of the nature of the coalition's objective, its primary strategy was to lobby the state legislature. Realizing that the impact is stronger when coalitions present a united front, the group chose to address issues on which the four organizations agreed, and not to discuss matters on which they disagreed.

Actions

The coalition chose to be informal, with two representatives from each group constituting a steering committee. They contracted with a professional lobbyist for assistance in planning their legislative agenda. The lobbyist ensured that the coalition had access to the political power structure not only during the legislative session, but prior to the introduction of specific legislation. The coalition also turned to professional organizations and others for additional research and assistance.

Before any lobbying, which was the principle activity, members planned and rehearsed their presentations together.

The coalition drafted a bill that would require the state health department to prepare a five-year plan to identify and meet the needs of mentally ill adults. It also initiated two patients' rights bills and inspired two other measures: one to expand community treatment and residential services for emotionally handicapped children and adolescents; the other to establish a commission on the future of state psychiatric hospitals.

Outcome

Between 1985 and 1988, Maryland appropriations for community treatment, and rehabilitative, residential and other services for adults with long-term disabling mental illness increased by more than $15 million. These funds helped finance 1,000 new community housing placements and 1,800 new psychosocial rehabilitation placements. Maryland's total community health budget increased from $20.4 million at the end of 1983 to $55.2 million by 1988. A large portion of this increase was used for citizens with long term illnesses, as the coalition advocated. In addition to these dramatic budgetary shifts, the following legislative developments took place:

- A bill requiring a state five-year plan on the needs of mentally ill adults was passed in 1984.
- Patients' rights bills were enacted in 1985.
- Bills to expand community treatment and residential services, and to set up a study commission on psychiatric hospitals, were passed in 1986.
- Collaboration between citizens' organizations and mental health professional societies resulted in legislation raising health insurance benefits for outpatient treatment of mental illnesses from 50 to 60 percent of the benefits provided for other illnesses.

Evaluation

A coalition composed of independent statewide organizations can induce increased state funding for treatment of the mentally ill and their families through
unified action. This case illustrates the importance of a coalition that presents a
strong, unified public and political image—avoiding public disagreements, which
can be extremely damaging. This coalition drew additional energy by including in
its effort those directly affected by the outcome: mentally ill citizens and former
residents of psychiatric facilities.

Analysis of tactics

The following tactics were used (not necessarily in this order). See "Advocacy Tactics," Chapter 7, for more information.

Tactic 1   Conduct studies of the issue
Tactic 23   Lobby decision-makers
Tactic 32   Seek enactment of new laws, policies or regulations

Case 4
The polluting incinerators

The problem

Industrial incinerators in Mitchell and Caldwell counties, North Carolina, operated in violation of state law, arousing citizen complaints and threatening their
health and that of the environment.

The issue

To agitate for the closure of facilities that failed to comply with the law.

There are two case histories that concern this issue, one in each of the counties
affected, so we will describe them each in turn.

A. Mitchell County

Background

Despite a four-year history that included citizen complaints and citations by a state
agency against Mitchell Systems, operator of an industrial incinerator, it appeared in

1985 that the firm would get final approval for expanded waste disposal in Mitchell County. This state of affairs was particularly galling because, two years earlier, the North Carolina Department of Natural Resources and Community Development (NRCD) determined that Mitchell Systems' owner had falsified a 1980 permit application, building an incinerator much larger than the 1,800 pound-per-hour facility he sought on paper. The NRCD informed the owner in May, 1983 that he could not expand his operations until he applied for an amended permit.

The owner, Mr. Foushee, was not new to the waste business, owning a similar enterprise, Caldwell Systems, in neighboring Caldwell County (see below). He was also a gubernatorial appointee of the state Hazardous Waste Treatment Commission, which oversees construction of hazardous waste facilities.

From the beginning, the Mitchell County facility was the target of continuous complaints from nearby residents. Neighbors said that heavy black smoke, with flames up to fifty feet high, caused choking odors and eye irritation, at times severe enough to make work impossible. In addition, they had observed trucks entering the plant without placards identifying the chemicals being transported, as required by law.

In response to the complaints, NRCD began periodic inspections of the facility in 1981. The agency issued a number of citations over the next two years. Violations included: traces of organic and heavy metal contamination of soil; recurrent improper temperature gauge operation and opacity measurements; inadequate hazardous waste combustion; and the use of waste oil, rather than natural gas as specified in the NRCD permit, for fueling the second burner. Also, Mitchell Systems failed to submit lists of hazardous waste burned in 1981 and 1982.

By 1985 Mitchell Systems had yet to be fined or penalized for any violation. Its final waste permit appeared inevitable.

The advocate group and its objective

Citizens for a Safe Environment was formed in 1985, with the aim of driving Mitchell Systems from the community.

Strategy

Advocates undertook a broad plan for gathering evidence demonstrating the hazardous nature of the Mitchell Systems operation. This included setting up a citizens' watch for permit violations, and joining with other groups that could help in the effort.

Actions

By the time Citizens for a Safe Environment was formed, there was already a substantial history of citizens' complaints, NRCD citations, and other actions that had increased pressure on the waste plant. Among them:

- Bruce Biddix, newly returned to his home in Mitchell County after twenty one years in the Coast Guard, conducted a petition drive against the plant's application for expansion, obtaining 2,000 signatures. While state officials did not react overtly to Biddix' effort, the petition left no doubt about popular opposition to the plant, and heightened the problem's visibility.

- Four former Mitchell Systems employees provided affidavits detailing unsafe conditions at the plant, an action that led to a videotape documenting the conditions and an article in the Durham paper, the *Independent*.

- The Mitchell County Commission appointed a Citizen's Advisory Board on Hazardous Waste to protect citizen concerns during the permit process. The board obtained a $15,000 grant to hire consultants for its work.

- The Mitchell County Chapter of the Western North Carolina Alliance, formed in April 1985, began a letter-writing campaign criticizing Governor Jim Martin for appointing Mr. Foushee to the state Hazardous Waste Treatment Commission. Three Mitchell County commissioners also visited Governor Martin, seeking Foushee's removal from the commission.

In addition to developing evidence against Mitchell Systems, Citizens for a Safe Environment maintained a publicity campaign on the issue, and developed allies in other communities. Members also helped with data collection, which involved conducting a community health survey, interviewing former Mitchell Systems' employees, investigating the incinerator's impact on property values, and examining violations of hazardous-waste haulers.

In July, 1985, Mitchell Systems' environmental insurance lapsed and was not renewed. The Hazardous Waste Branch of the Department of Human Resources fined the company $107 per day of operation without insurance. Foushee appealed, but eventually paid the fine and obtained new insurance.

In December, 1985, landowners brought two civil suits against Mitchell Systems, citing loss of property value and other damages.

Outcome

- While the Mitchell County commissioners' request for the plant owner's removal from the Hazardous Waste Treatment Commission was rejected initially, he resigned soon thereafter.

- The Hazardous Waste Branch informed Foushee in the fall of 1985 of more than 200 violations of his permit and gave him until January 24, 1986, to correct them. On January 24, Foushee announced Mitchell Systems was closing due to economic failure.

- Through organized and compelling testimony, advocates achieved satisfactory revisions of the plant closure plan. Witnesses included Marshall Hale, a former employee at the incinerator, and his wife, Betty. Hale suffered from neurological damage and other complications he felt could be traced to his work at Mitchell Systems. The county pledged to follow a plan that would include on- and off-site sampling for environmental contaminants, including continuing studies of soil and water.

- Mitchell County advocates became a regional resource for other communities concerned about health factors related to industrial incinerators. They advised others about combating similar targets, including Foushee's plant in Caldwell County.

B. Caldwell County

The Advocate Group and its Objective

Caldwell Concerned Citizens for a Clean Environment (4CE) formed to determine whether the waste disposal facility in their county, Caldwell Systems (also owned by Foushee) posed a health problem.

Strategy

4CE researched the necessary data about Caldwell Systems. They developed alternative ways to achieve their objective, and planned various ways to apply pressure on uncooperative regulatory bodies.

Actions

Equipped with campaign brochures describing incinerator problems, 4CE proposed off-site testing to state officials, but were turned down. They undertook their own tests, which revealed significant contamination. Presented with this damning evidence, the state started to investigate, as statewide media were beginning to question North Carolina's ability to regulate such facilities.

County hearings were held, at which Caldwell Systems came under increasing pressure. A local physician, Marc Guerra, testified at the hearings that the incinerator threatened the health of residents and workers at the plant. At the recommendation of the study committee, the county commissioners called for the eviction of Caldwell Systems.

Foushee threatened legal action, then attempted to bargain for continued waste treatment and storage at the site in return for the immediate cessation of burning. At this point the commissioners, negotiating on behalf of the county, deferred to 4CE (which had by now developed considerable influence) on whether to compromise or sue Foushee. 4CE elected to settle, provided the county would pay the sum of $99,000 to a local dairy farmer whose land had been contaminated by the plant.

Outcome

Numerous legal battles continued with respect to the Caldwell Systems' operation, as local advocates monitored the facility. Like their counterparts in Mitchell County, members of 4CE also began serving as resources for other communities that were threatened .

Evaluation

Well-organized community coalitions can terminate the corrupt business of an established community leader or bring it to heel. There were many important ingredients in the Mitchell and Caldwell counties' campaigns. In the opinion of observers, the communities' health was protected without compromise thanks to the following factors:

- Steadily mounting pressure on the target;
- Evidence from testimony and testing;
- The expertise of those gathering data and dealing with regulators;
- An understanding about the gravity of the matter by local officials.

In addition, there was great persistence on the part of the advocates — as demonstrated by the way 4CE developed an alternative plan for off-site contamination tests when it was rebuffed by established channels. The strong evidence resulting from this testing forced state action, which put the crucial squeeze on the offending plant.

Bruce Biddix personified persistence in Mitchell County. Besides his petition drive, he was a one-man monitoring agency, often spending cold nights on guard to guarantee that trucks were not violating the state's order prohibiting Mitchell Systems from accepting waste.

There was also extensive media attention, which can strengthen a campaign by lending it legitimacy, as it did here. Such positive attention not only heightens public awareness of a problem and extends opposition to it, but frequently emboldens advocates and raises the tide of change.

There were other dramatic factors whose impact cannot easily be measured, including the fact that citizens and professionals were willing to step forward and testify against the plants.

Analysis of Tactics

The following tactics were included (not necessarily in this order). See "Advocacy Tactics," Chapter 7, for more information.

Tactic 6   Document complaints
Tactic 7   Act as a watchdog
Tactic 20   Express opposition publicly
Tactic 26   Conduct a petition drive
Tactic 30   File a formal complaint
Tactic 31   Seek enforcement of existing laws, policies or regulations
Tactic 32   Seek enactment of new laws, policies or regulations
Tactic 36   Initiate legal action
Tactic 37   Arrange a media exposé

Case 5
Health care for the poor in Arkansas

The problem

Health care was unavailable to the poor of Lee County, Arkansas.

The issue

To determine the major health needs of Lee County and devise and implement ways to meet them.

Background

Activists in Lee County, Arkansas, and the Volunteers in Service to America program (VISTA) came together in 1969 to help alleviate conditions in this flatland area 120 miles east of Little Rock and seventy miles southeast of Memphis. More than half of the 18,000 inhabitants in this 200-square-mile area were black and poor.

Help came in the form of federal legislation establishing the Office of Economic Opportunity (OEO), the governing agency of VISTA. One of their aims was empowering the poor. In Lee County, VISTA found many elements of the Old South untouched by time. Segregation and plantations with adjacent wooden shacks, inhabited by black field hands, were commonplace. Local government was all white. Many homes of blacks were accessible only by dirt roads, and few had indoor plumbing.

The poor had virtually no access to health care. The physician-to-population ratio was 20 percent that of the national average. Lee Memorial Hospital, the local hospital, had only 25 beds. The county health department consisted of two under-qualified employees, and the nearest clinic that accepted "charity cases" was in Memphis, seventy miles away.

The advocate group and its objective

The VISTA volunteers organized four Neighborhood Action Councils (NACs). NAC representatives were recruited door-to-door and by means of church announcements and store window signs.

Their objective was to develop a community-controlled clinic. VISTA concluded that community-control was important for several reasons:
1. The rural poor understood their own needs, and they would call for the development of appropriate services.
2. Although generations of Lee County's poor blacks had depended on the charity of affluent whites, like other oppressed groups they could transcend poverty, submission and dependence by seizing control of their lives.
3. A community-controlled clinic might serve as a model organization that could inspire collective action in other areas and, at the same time, provide further impetus for empowerment of the poor.

Actions

In a series of meetings, NAC recruits were invited to discuss local problems, especially health problems.

From the outset, the NACs agreed about the primary health problem: the absence of health care for the poor. Each NAC elected two representatives to the board of the proposed Lee County Cooperative Clinic. The board applied for an OEO operating grant.

Even as the application was pending, the board raised $2,000 through community projects, and VISTA opened a "mini-clinic" in a car belonging to one of the physician volunteers, Dan Blumenthal. In an effort to expand beyond the facilities of-fered by his car, and gain access to Lee Memorial Hospital, Blumenthal applied for membership in the Lee County Medical Society. To back him up, the directors of the Lee County Cooperative Clinic appointed a committee to negotiate with the medical society and the hospital to gain access for clinic doctors to the hospital's facilities. Those negotiations failed, and the clinic filed a class action suit in federal court to gain access. In addition, three of the directors and three VISTA volunteers went to Washington to lobby OEO for clinic funding.

The dispute attracted the attention of some of the national news media, but the additional publicity further polarized the community and the clinic advocates.

Outcome

Opposition to VISTA and the proposed clinic steadily mounted as the struggle moved into court and onto the national forum. Vocal opponents included numer-ous white community leaders, such as the minister of the First Baptist Church, and shop and plantation owners.

In December, 1969, however, OEO granted nearly $40,000 for the clinic. It opened in March, 1970, with a staff of seven employees from the community, and seven VISTA volunteers. Later, funding was to increase; in 1972, OEO approved a $1.2 million funding request for the clinic to expand. Local opponents, with the support of the governor of the state, made an attempt to block the grant. A com-promise devised by the governor and accepted by both sides added five new white members to the board, but the white opposition remained a minority.

The Lee County Cooperative Clinic served as a rallying point for raising self-re-spect within the black poor community. Throughout the struggle, the black com-munity grew stronger, forming political organizations and conducting boycotts in the early 1970s. However, many factors worked against maintaining a clinic with comprehensive services over the long term. Recruiting and maintaining physi-cians at wages and benefits far below the potential existing elsewhere was a con-tinuing problem. As the government funding it relied on diminished, the clinic made proportionate reductions in its comprehensive services.

Evaluation

A well-organized outside group can help empower a poor community to work for political and social change by establishing a community-controlled health care organization.

As in other campaigns, it was important in Lee County that the local community establish control of the organization from the outset. Local directors were better equipped than outsiders to make crucial decision affecting the organization's future. For example, the clinic board stood up to the governor's threats to expansion, because the directors were tied intimately to the whole struggle.

Analysis of Tactics

The following tactics were used (not necessarily in this order). See "Advocacy Tactics," Chapter 7, for more information.

Tactic 11   Develop proposals

Tactic 14   Offer public education

Tactic 17   Establish an alternative system or program

Tactic 36   Initiate legal action

Appendix A

Power Structure Research

Here you will find more information on the techniques of power structure research mentioned in Chapter 3: "Understanding the Issue."

Power structure research is one example of root cause analysis, which was discussed in Chapter 3. It may be more complicated and controversial than other methods discussed in this handbook; you should consider carefully whether you want to apply this method to your issue. The potential pitfalls are obvious: it may be all too easy to put the opposition on the defensive too early, before you are ready. However, for some groups and for some issues, power structure research provides the best way to determine root causes and points for intervention.

Power structure research starts with two questions:
- Who is responsible for the problem?
- Who has the power to solve it?

There are three well-established steps you can take to answer those questions:
1. Identify the relevant information infrastructure;
2. Crack the information bank;
3. Having identified the power, go straight to it for information.

1. Identify the relevant information infrastructure

Ties between institutions and modern technology produce a steady flow of accurate data on virtually every aspect of human behavior. For each sector of society, there is an information infrastructure. It may be in government agencies, university research centers, professional organizations, trade associations, special libraries, or companies that publish trade books, periodicals and newspapers. Numerous reference books availabile in libraries help identify the information infrastructure, including the *United States Government Organization Manual*, the *Encyclopedia of Associations*, the *Research Centers Directory*, the *Foundation Directory*, the *Directory of Special Libraries and Information Centers*, and the *Directory of National Trade and Professional Associations in the United States*.

2. Crack the information bank

Having identified relevant sources, the next step is accessing information to determine your issue's key players. U.S. citizens have legal access to vast banks of public documents and data. Some simple techniques can improve your chances of gaining the requested data in a timely fashion. Examples include the use of printed stationery, which makes your request look professional; telephoning, until you can pinpoint the right person for a request; familiarizing yourself with relevant professional jargon; or developing contacts on the inside. Here are some ways to gain insight into the workings of corporations, law firms, individuals and affiliations, elected officials, property owners, lobbyists and government officials.

A. Major corporations

Investigative forays into corporations invariably lead with several basic questions (see Collette: *Research Guide for Leaders*), including:
1. Who owns and controls the company?
2. Who are the officers and directors, and what are their interlocking directorates?
3. What are the money flow and financial relationships between them?
4. What problems has the company experienced?

Annual reports provide the company's view of its history, management, financial condition, plant locations and future plans. Biased though annual reports they may be, there are facts to be gleaned from them. Publicly held corporations must file numerous reports with the Securities and Exchange Commission, including Form 10-K, Form 8-K, a proxy statement, and Form 13-F. They are prime sources of information about the firm's stock ownership; its directors and executive officers, including their wealth and holdings; money flow; pending legal proceedings; mergers and acquisitions; changes in control or assets; and major institutional stockholders.

There are a variety of directories available in public libraries that describe the directors, officers and interlocking relationships. Examples are Standard and Poor's *Register of Corporations, Directors and Executives* and Dun & Bradstreet's *Middle Market Directory*. Investment guides, such as *Value Line's Investment Survey and* Moody's *Banking and Finance Manual* give you information about stock ownership and control.

Court records from actions where corporations have been plaintiffs or defendants can be a veritable gold mine of information, whether through documents that were admitted as evidence, or from the trial's record of testimony. Other state and local records, such as tax assessment records, may contain useful information about the firm, its managers, lawyers, allies and enemies.

Still other resources, such as Standard and Poor's *Corporation Records*, provide more detailed descriptions of many companies' production and financial structure.

B. Law firms

Many politicians, lobbyists and decision-makers are lawyers. The Martindale-Hubbell *Law Directory* gives information on all lawyers and most law firms in the country, including biographical data, a partial listing of corporate clients, and often financial worth.

C. Individuals and their affiliations

Who's Who directories for almost every vocation, location and minority present a range of information, including biographical data, corporate involvements, and past political relationships. Research can determine a range of affiliations from both *Who's Who* directories and the *Foundation Directory*. These would indicate ties between corporations; between law firms and corporations; between foundations and the web of banks, corporations, and non-profits.

Court records will state whether a person has ever been arrested, sued or had judgments against him or her, as well as whether the subject has ever had anyone else arrested or sued. Tax records show what real estate a person owns, the assessed value of the property, improvements on the property and delinquent taxes. For more specific guidance, see D. Noyes' *Raising Hell*.

D. Elected officials

"To understand politicians, you need to follow the money" (Noyes, 1983). The ethics statement, also known in some locations as a "statement of economic interests," lists a politician's income from outside sources, such as stock dividends, consulting fees, income from speaking engagements, and sales commissions.

Campaign reporting forms give expense records of campaigns. Voting records are also public information. Common Cause, a public interest advocacy organization, examines such records to see if there are any links between elected officials' major campaign contributors and their voting records.

E. Property owners

Local property and/or tax documents, which are public records on file with local governmental agencies, provide information about property owners.

F. Lobbyists

Major interest groups, including corporations, trade associations, churches, labor organizations and citizens groups, employ people to lobby for them at city hall, the state capital and Congress. Lobbyists must register in most states with the secretary of state.

G. Non-elected government officials

The U.S. Civil Service Commission, the *Federal Yellow Book* and the *National Directory of State Agencies* show how various governmental offices, branches and bureaus are organized. The *Congressional Directory* provides basic background information about the staffs of elected officials.

3. Having identified the power, go straight to it for information

Who but decision-makers can offer as much information about decision-makers? Interviewing them can be very informative. This is often the case even if they're engaged in subterfuge, because when we spot camouflage or denial we can often tap into some of the target's major weaknesses. You will invariably find rewards when you come to such interviews prepared, knowing as much as possible about the individual, his or her organization, and the topic of interest.

As you will find, revealing all that you know will not necessarily help you achieve the goal of gaining more information. Indeed, attempts to dazzle the targets with the extent of your knowledge are likely to put them on the defensive, which may lead to stonewalling, or a series of misleading statements. The best approach is one that will ensure, to the extent possible, the comfort of your subject. To this end, it's useful to open with small talk as you and the subject seek common ground and, hence, a comfort zone. You're not co-opting your principles, but preserving this opportunity to gain potentially vital information—to learn by listening, or to lead the conversation where you want it to go.

Appendix B

Framing the Issue

The following presentation represents one way of framing an issue — in this case, the effects of smoking. See page 61 of Chapter 7, "Advocacy Tactics," for more information.

This presentation was used by the North Bay Health Resources Center in California to motivate teens to work on tobacco issues (Records & Altman, 1992). It is now used throughout California.

The BB Demonstration

For this demonstration, you will need a large metal canning or cooking kettle. The demonstration relies on the dramatic sound of hundreds of BBs falling into the kettle. That sound will be enhanced if you put a metal lid inside it, resting on a glass or cup to make a good sounding board—otherwise the first BBs you throw in your kettle will muffle the sound of later ones. (If you want the sound to be deafening, use a microphone and amplifier.)

Before you start, put the indicated number of BBs in labeled jars, as follows:

1	Start-up
16	Hard drugs
342	Alcohol
1,180	Tobacco (1,323, if you want to include environmental figures)

Time-saving tip

If you plan to do this demonstration more than once, draw a line on the "alcohol" and "tobacco" jars after you have counted out the appropriate number of BBs. For future demonstrations, simply fill to the line.

Presentation tip

Timing is important for this demonstration. If you pour the BBs too fast, or too slowly, you will lose some of the impact.

The Presentation

Begin by saying: "We all know tobacco is harmful to our health, but few of us really understand just how harmful it is. To give you a new perspective on the problem of tobacco, I'm going to ask you to think about death.

"I have a metal BB here. Now listen to the sound it makes when I throw it in this kettle."

Toss BB into kettle, say: "Let the sound of one BB..."

Toss second BB into kettle: "...represent one death. Think about someone you know who died.

"First, let's think for a moment about hard drugs—cocaine (which includes crack) and heroin. You think they're bad? They are. They'll kill you ... Here's how many people will die from a drug overdose every day in this country..."

Pour 16 BBs slowly: "That represents sixteen people who will die every day from these drugs—about 5,700 people every year.

"Now what about alcohol? Do you think alcohol is bad for you? It is. It will kill you. Usually not right away, but slowly over time. Here's how many people will die from alcohol every day..."

Pour 342 BBs slowly: "That's 342 people every day, 125,000 every year.

Pour slowly, pause: "Now tobacco—listen to how many people tobacco will kill today and every day in this country..."

Pour remaining BBs: "That's 1,180 people who die every day and are dying right now—430,000 people every year. (If you want to include people who die from environmental tobacco smoke, the total would be 483,000 people who die each year: 1,323 per day).

"Three out of four people who are dying from tobacco today and every day started to smoke before they were eighteen years old. About half started before they were thirteen years old.

"Tobacco kills. It won't kill today, or tomorrow like hard drugs can. But think about this. The tobacco industry must recruit 5,000 new smokers every day to replace those who have quit or died. And they're trying to recruit kids.

"Remember, tobacco is the only legal consumer product in the United States today that, when used as intended, will kill you."

For presentations at schools, you can conclude with: "So don't be a BB, and don't let your family or friends be BBs either."

References

Ahmed, K. 1991. *Good works: A guide to careers in social change. 4th edition.* New York: Barricade Books.

Alinsky, S.D. 1971. *Rules for radicals.* New York: Vintage Books.

Bobo, K., Kendall, J., and Max, S. 1991. *Organizing for social change: A manual for activists in the 1990s.* Washington, D.C.: Seven Locks Press.

Boston Urban Study Group. 1984. *Who rules Boston? A citizen's guide to reclaiming the city.* Boston: The Institute for Democratic Socialism.

Collette, W. 1987. *Research guide for leaders.* Arlington, Va.: Citizen's Clearinghouse for Hazardous Waste, Inc.

Dale, D. 1978. *How to make citizen involvement work.* Amherst, Mass.: Citizen Involvement Training Project.

De Tocqueville, A. 1835. *Democracy in America.*

Douglas, C., and Claypoole, J. 1992. *Why policy?* Presentation made at the ASSIST training, October 14, Washington, D.C.

Farren, Pat, ed. 1991. *A way of life: Celebrating sustained activism, Peace Calendar, Volume 36.* New York: War Resisters League, and Philadelphia: New Society Publishers.

Fawcett, S.B., Paine, A.L., Francisco, V.T., and Vliet, M. 1993. Promoting health through community development. In D. Glenwick & L.A. Jason (eds.), *Promoting health and mental health in children, youth, and families.* New York: Springer Publishing.

Fawcett, S.B., Seekins, T., and Jason, L.A. 1987. Policy research and child passenger safety legislation: A case study and experimental evaluation. *Journal of Social Issues,* 43, 133-148.

Furniss, E. S., Jr. 1966. *Counterinsurgency: Some problems and implications.* New York: Council on Religion and International Affairs.

Futurist and *Future Survey.* World Future Society: Washington, D.C.

Holland, J., and Henriot, P. 1988. *Social analysis: Linking faith and justice.* Washington, D.C.: Center of Concern.

Hope, A., and Timmel, S. 1984. *Training for transformation: A handbook for communty workers.* Zimbabwe: Mambo Press.

Kahn, S. 1982. *Organizing.* New York: McGraw Hill.

Legator, M.S., Harper, B.L., and Scott, M.J. 1985. *The health detective's handbook*. Baltimore: The Johns Hopkins University Press.

Liddell Hart, B.H. 1944. *Thoughts on war*. London: Faber and Faber.

Mayer, R.N. 1989. *The consumer movement*. Boston: Twayne Publishers.

Mayster, V., Waitzkin, H., Hubbell, F.A., and Rucker, L. 1990. Local advocacy for the medically indigent. *Journal of the American Medical Association*, 263 (2), 262-268.

Nader, R. Updated edition: 1972. *Unsafe at any speed: The design-in dangers of the American automobile*. New York: Grossman.

Noyes, D. 1983. Raising hell: A citizens guide to the fine art of investigation. San Francisco: *Mother Jones Magazine*.

Records, J., and Altman, D. G. 1992. Tobacco and kids: Using creative epidemiology to move an audience. *Tobacco Control* 1 (1) p. 59.

Sharp, G. 1973. *The politics of nonviolent action*. Boston: Extending Horizons Books.

Speeter, G. 1978. *Power: A repossession manual*. Amherst, Mass.: Citizen Involvement Training Project.

Staples, L. 1984. *Roots to power*. New York: Praeger.

Swords, P. 1991. Advocacy without fear. *The Grantsmanship Center Whole Nonprofit Catalog* (summer), page 20.

United Way of America. 1989. *What lies ahead: Countdown to the 21st Century*. Alexandria, Va.: United Way Strategic Institute.

Weiner, L. 1994. *Media Advocacy for Tobacco Control*. Stanford Calif.: Health Promotion Resource Center, for California Department of Health Services, Tobacco Control Section.

Werner, D., and Bower, B. 1982. *Helping health workers learn*. Palo Alto, Calif.: The Hesperian Foundation.

Zander, A. 1990. *Effective social action by community groups*. San Francisco: Jossey-Bass.

Additional Resources

How-to Guides

A modular system of short guides developed in 1989-93 for the use of health promotion professionals and grassroots organizers. For more information, write: Distribution, Health Promotion Resource Center, Stanford Center for Research in Disease Prevention
1000 Welch Road, Palo Alto, CA 94304-1885
Tel: (415) 723-0003

Titles include:
Building and Maintaining Effective Coalitions
Conducting a Community Resource Inventory
Finding the Information You Need
Focus Groups
Gaining Access to Media Resources
Holding Press Conferences
How to Hire and Use a Consultant
Preparing for Media Interviews
Running Effective Meetings
Teambuilding for Community Health Promotion
Volunteers
Working with Media Gatekeepers
Writing and Sending Press Releases
Writing Effective Survey Questions

Media

Media Advocacy and Public Health, by L. Wallack, L. Dorfman, D. Jernigan, et al. Sage Publications, Newbury Park, Calif. 1993.

Media Advocacy Training Handbook. The Marin Institute for the Prevention of Alcohol and Other Drug Problems, San Rafael, Calif. 1992.

Media Strategies for Smoking Control. Advocacy Institute, Washington, D.C. 1989

Smoke Signals. Advocacy Institute, Washington, D.C. 1989.

Evaluation

Evaluation: A Systematic Approach, by P. Rossi and H. Freeman. Sage Publications: Newbury Park, Calif. 1985.

Behavioral Risk Factor Surveys. Centers for Disease Control and Prevention, Mail Stop K30, 4770 Buford Highway, Atlanta, GA 30341-3724.

Evaluator's Handbook, by J. Herman and L. Morris. Sage Publications: Newbury Park, Calif. 1987.

Focus Groups: A Practical Guide for Applied Research, by Richard A. Krueger. Sage Publications: Newbury Park, Calif. 1988.

How to Design a Program Evaluation, by C. Fitz-Gibbon and L. Morris. Sage Publications: Newbury Park, Calif. 1987.

Program Evaluation Kit, 2nd Ed., by J. Herman. Sage Publications: Newbury Park, Calif. 1988.

Youth Risk Behavior Survey. Centers for Disease Control and Prevention, Mail Stop K33, 4770 Buford Highway, Atlanta, GA 30341-3724.

Leadership

Leaders, by B. Nanus and LW. Bennis. Harper and Row, New York. 1985.

Leadership is an Art, by M. De Pree. Dell Publishing, New York. 1989.

Why Leaders Can't Lead, by W. Bennis. Jossey-Bass, San Francisco. 1989.